What a great addition to the counselling toolkit! At last, a book that not only recognizes the therapeutic value of exploring one's family history, but also provides detailed instructions to mental health practitioners for how to conduct these explorations in group settings. In clear and accessible language, the authors explain their "Legacy Model" approach to wellness, sensitively employing case material to illustrate how it works. Their approach, while designed for older adults, could be adapted for any age group. Highly recommended.

– **Susan Moore, PhD**, *Emeritus Professor, Swinburne University of Technology, Australia*

Bacon, Anderson & Boiros have crafted a comprehensive text for group workers using the Legacy Model to enhance psychological wellness with veterans and older adults. The authors offer useful examples of project ideas, moving memoirs and multiple resources for clinicians. A great contribution to group work!

– **Ana Puig, PhD**, *Professor, University of Florida and Past President of the Association for Specialists in Group Work*

CONDUCTING WELLNESS GROUPS FOR VETERANS AND OLDER ADULTS

Conducting Wellness Groups for Veterans and Older Adults: The Legacy Model offers an innovative wellness group model for mental health practitioners. Two curricula developed by the authors are explored: the Process-Focused Legacy Group curriculum for members who are high-functioning and motivated adults and the Activity-Based Legacy Group curriculum tailored for persons with disabilities and/or cognitive impairments. Detailed steps, prompts, and legacy activities are provided for each stage for both curriculum formats. This book provides clinical examples from the facilitator's group experiences using the Legacy Model. The appendices provide further detailed resource materials that include descriptions of potential legacy projects and a vast assortment of legacy activities.

This book is essential for mental health practitioners: mental health counselors, marriage and family therapists, social workers, and psychologists interested in conducting Legacy Groups with veterans and older adults.

Dr. Victoria L. Bacon, CGP, is a licensed psychologist and internationally certified group psychotherapist who has created, taught, and conducted groups with 40 years' experience teaching, presenting, and providing workshops.

Dr. Kristen E. Anderson, LCPC, is a mental health and substance abuse counselor in private practice, Chicago, Illinois. She has extensive experience in individual and group counseling, specializing in neurofeedback.

Maureen F. Boiros, MEd, RN, is a mental health counselor and certified peer specialist who conducts groups for spouses of combat veterans and has experience as a nurse working with developmentally disabled adults.

CONDUCTING WELLNESS GROUPS FOR VETERANS AND OLDER ADULTS

The Legacy Model

Victoria L. Bacon, Kristen E. Anderson
and Maureen F. Boiros

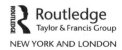

Routledge
Taylor & Francis Group

NEW YORK AND LONDON

Cover image: From Getty

First published 2023
by Routledge
605 Third Avenue, New York, NY 10158

and by Routledge
4 Park Square, Milton Park, Abingdon, Oxon, OX14 4RN

Routledge is an imprint of the Taylor & Francis Group, an informa business

© 2023 Victoria L. Bacon, Kristen E. Anderson, and Maureen F. Boiros

The right of Victoria L. Bacon, Kristen E. Anderson, and Maureen
F. Boiros to be identified as authors of this work has been asserted in
accordance with sections 77 and 78 of the Copyright, Designs and
Patents Act 1988.

All rights reserved. No part of this book may be reprinted or reproduced
or utilised in any form or by any electronic, mechanical, or other
means, now known or hereafter invented, including photocopying and
recording, or in any information storage or retrieval system, without
permission in writing from the publishers.

Trademark notice: Product or corporate names may be trademarks or
registered trademarks, and are used only for identification and explanation
without intent to infringe.

Library of Congress Cataloging-in-Publication Data
Names: Bacon, Victoria L., author. | Anderson, Kristen E., author. |
   Boiros, Maureen F., author.
Title: Conducting wellness groups for veterans and older adults :
   the legacy model / Victoria L. Bacon, Kristen E. Anderson,
   Maureen F. Boiros.
Description: New York, NY : Routledge, 2022. | Includes
   bibliographical references and index. | Identifiers: LCCN 2022015066
   (print) | LCCN 2022015067 (ebook) | ISBN 9781032287102
   (hardback) | ISBN 9781032286655 (paperback) |
   ISBN 9781003298168 (ebook)
Subjects: LCSH: Group psychotherapy. | Group psychotherapy for
   older people. | Group counseling. | Older people—Mental health. |
   Veterans—Mental health. | Intergenerational relations—Psychological
   aspects.
Classification: LCC RC488 .B314 2022 (print) | LCC RC488 (ebook) |
   DDC 616.89/152—dc23/eng/20220523
LC record available at https://lccn.loc.gov/2022015066
LC ebook record available at https://lccn.loc.gov/2022015067

ISBN: 978-1-032-28710-2 (hbk)
ISBN: 978-1-032-28665-5 (pbk)
ISBN: 978-1-003-29816-8 (ebk)

DOI: 10.4324/9781003298168

Typeset in Bembo
by Apex CoVantage, LLC

Access the Support Material: www.routledge.com/9781032286655

Dedicated to the healing power of legacy.

CONTENTS

PREFACE

The story began on December 20, 1996, when I attended a holiday party in New Hampshire. The usual friends were there, including Mickey, a high-spirited, talkative man, who had just become a father. He was taking fatherhood rather seriously and, therefore, decided to explore his family history. Mickey wanted to give the gift of his legacy to his firstborn child. This involved genealogy research that he was conducting in New Hampshire and Massachusetts, as this material was not widely available on the internet. I was so engrossed with listening to him about his research efforts that I hardly spoke to my other friends. Mickey invited me to meet him at the National Archives in Waltham, Massachusetts, so he could walk me through the research process. At first, I was hesitant, as my father was an orphan and my mother had died when I was young, leaving me very little family history to begin genealogy research. I did share with Mickey that I had been very fond of my maternal grandmother and her family history was a mystery as no living relative knew her story. I did finally agree to meet him. This began my journey into my family legacy.

As the journey began in earnest, many challenges surfaced in my research, including just having accepted a full-time teaching position at a university. Academic life left little time for personal research. A few key highlights along my path over these years include connecting with a cousin once removed, meeting or being reunited with my mother's living siblings, reuniting with a cousin, receiving family photos from relatives, and becoming a member of the Daughters of the American Revolution (DAR) on October 9, 2004. Visits to family cemetery plots have been an exciting and rewarding venture since 1996, uncovering a wealth of information and experiencing uncanny coincidences. More recently, I have met one of my father's orphan brothers and visited the farm that my father grew up on as a child and learned that I am a descendant of the Huguenots of

New Paltz, New York. In December 2014, my cousin Robin found my maternal grandmother's birth certificate online, as it had been just scanned and made available in the New Hampshire vital records, as this was the initial motivation for commencing the search for my family history and legacy.

In May 2012, several of my scholarly projects came to completion. I felt a great sense of accomplishment and an overwhelming sense of freedom. It was at this time that I decided to develop a Legacy Group Model. A group model had been in the back of my mind for many years culminating in writing an article in 2006 that was awarded the Women's Issues Writing Contest, Health Category, from the Massachusetts DAR. It was not until 2012 did I mention the Legacy Group idea and project to my dean, as I wanted to apply for grant money. With a green light, the project was officially launched in April 2013 with a Special Projects Grant from the DAR and Bridgewater State University (BSU) matching funds. In addition, the College of Graduate Studies provided a graduate assistant to work on this research and community service project. I then contacted BSU alumni who had stood apart as graduate students and were mental health practitioners to form a team for the project. Kristen E. Anderson and Melissa Shea jumped on board. Maureen F. Boiros was completing her last year of her graduate program and served as the graduate research assistant during the first year of the project. She was a retired registered nurse and decided to get formally trained as a mental health counselor to work with veterans. Once she graduated with her master's degree, she seamlessly transitioned to colleague. Melissa Shea served as a group facilitator, mentor, and creative genius. Unfortunately, she was not able to work on the manuscript due to caretaking responsibilities. During this time, Kristen E. Anderson completed a doctoral degree in gerontology and brought strong research and writing skills to the team.

The first Legacy Groups were conducted in 2013–2014 with women veterans at BSU. The rest is history.

Victoria L. Bacon

ACKNOWLEDGMENTS

We would like to thank our funding sources for their generosity and support of the multiyear research and community service Legacy Project. Foremost is Bridgewater State University (BSU) for awarding a Presidential Fellowship as well as grants from the Center for the Advancement of Research and Scholarship and the National Daughters of the American Revolution for a Special Projects Grant, especially Gail Terry, that funded the pilot program and for the Rotary Club of the Bridgewater Scholarship Grant monies. Thanks to the College of Graduate Studies at BSU for the following Graduate Research Assistants: Maureen F. Boiros, Shannon Delpapa, Mary Kate Bradley (Collins), and Kristina Walsh. We are grateful to the Office of Grants and Sponsored Projects, the support of BSU librarians, Tracy Charbonnier for creating the Legacy Project website, and Rena Arcao-McPhee for her work on the project.

We are grateful to the Veterans Service officers in Southeastern Massachusetts for getting the word out and to Andrew Boisvert of the Old Colony Historical Society of Taunton for the invaluable training workshop on conducting genealogical research. Jennifer Paley Parker for creating the Legacy Model logo and Dr. Carol Ryff for sharing the Ryff instrument and support materials. Thanks to Dr. Nikki Freeburg for reviewing our research methods.

Many thanks to Dean Lisa Battaglino and Provost Howard London for saying yes to the Legacy Project when it was in the idea stage. Much appreciation to President Dana-Mohler Faria for his support in awarding a Presidential Fellowship, which served as great momentum for the project. Deep gratitude to Dr. Marcia K. Anderson for her time and expertise in preparing the manuscript for publication. Our biggest thank you goes to Melissa Shea, our esteemed Legacy Group colleague. We thank her for her time, her creativity, and her talent.

Most importantly, our deep gratitude to the women veterans and older adults who allowed us the privilege of working with them in Legacy Groups.

INTRODUCTION

This book is divided into two parts. *Part I: Legacy Model Development* has four chapters to assist the readers in understanding how the Legacy Model was developed. Chapter 1, "Legacy Groups," introduces the concept of legacy and describes the Legacy Model. Chapter 2, "Theoretical Framework for the Legacy Model," reviews the key theories and concepts that were used to inform the development of the Model. Chapter 3, "Measuring the Effectiveness of the Legacy Model," provides an overview of the research study designed to assess the effectiveness of the Legacy Group curricula. The last chapter in this part, Chapter 4, "Serendipity in Legacy Work," explores serendipity, that is, uncanny coincidences that individuals may experience while exploring their legacy.

Part II: Legacy Group Curriculum in Action consists of four chapters and provides guidance and detailed steps for conducting Legacy Groups. Chapter 5, "Process-Focused Legacy Group Curriculum," provides an in-depth and step-by-step guidance on conducting Legacy Groups with high-functioning and motivated adults. Chapter 6, "Activity-Based Legacy Group Curriculum," is a curriculum for working with individuals with disabilities and/or cognitive challenges. This Legacy Group curriculum uses activities to encourage self-reflection and opportunities for members to complete the legacy projects during group sessions. Chapter 7, "Clinical Reflections," is devoted to reflections shared by group facilitators on the three types of groups they conducted: *Women Who Served*, *Adults in Search of Meaning*, and *Older Adults on a Journey*. Last, the book ends with Chapter 8, "Potential Audiences, Challenges, and Special Considerations," for practitioners interested in conducting Legacy Groups and Legacy Workshops with other populations as well as some best practice guidance.

The appendices provide useful information to facilitators who would like to learn about legacy exploration and preservation. Appendix I, Legacy Project Ideas, is a list of preservation projects as well as brief descriptions to share with group members. Appendix II, Legacy Group Resources, provides various resources to help prepare practitioners with facilitating Legacy Groups.

PART I

Legacy Model Development

Part I: Legacy Model Development has four chapters to assist the readers in. . . . . . .
understanding how the Legacy Model was developed. Chapter 1, "Legacy Groups,"
introduces the concept of legacy and describes the Legacy Model. Chapter 2,
"Theoretical Framework for the Legacy Model," reviews the key theories and
concepts that were used to inform the development of the Model. Chapter 3,
"Measuring the Effectiveness of the Legacy Model," provides an overview of
the research study designed to assess the effectiveness of the Legacy Group curricula. The last chapter in this section, Chapter 4, "Serendipity in Legacy Work,"
explores and normalizes serendipity, that is, uncanny coincidences that individuals
may experience while exploring their legacy.

Chapter 1 provides detailed information about the development of the Legacy
Model. The authors begin by defining legacy and then explain the purpose and
function of Legacy Groups. Chapter 2 delves into the theories and concepts
that are the theoretical underpinnings for this novel and innovative approach
for enhancing psychological wellness with veterans and older adults. Chapter 3
shares with the readers our research design and study findings from this multiyear
research and community service project. Chapter 4 explores serendipity, a topic
of great interest with individuals who engage in legacy work. As serendipitous
experiences, uncanny coincidences, are common, we hope to prepare facilitators
for these conversations.

DOI: 10.4324/9781003298168-1

PART II

Legacy Model Development

1
LEGACY GROUPS

Learning the benefits of a Legacy Group necessitates an understanding of what "legacy" encompasses and why individuals feel drawn to leave a legacy for those they care about. This chapter introduces the readers to the general concept of legacy, provides some ideas on how one might preserve their legacy, and explains how Legacy Groups are unique and an innovative group process while exploring one's legacy.

A Fifty-Year Silence by Miranda Richmond Mouillot (2015) details the author's quest to uncover the reason behind her grandparents' marital separation and ultimately her grandfather's refusal to ever speak her grandmother's name again. Her love for them both, and some sleuth work, drives the unveiling of their story and the events that led to their separation and silence. Significantly, through acquiring knowledge of her grandparent's stories, Mouillot gains a greater understanding of herself and how she engages in the world. The telling of their story offers Mouillot and the readers alike an exquisite account of the healing power of legacy.

Legacy Defined

You may be wondering, what are Legacy Groups? First, we need to gain a sense of the term "legacy." Bosak (2021), founder of the legacy project, states that "legacy is about life and living. It's about learning from the past, living in the present, and building for the future." Great people are known for leaving a legacy. A good example is Nelson Mandela, the first South African President, who left his legacy about fighting for civil rights. The Legacy Project contends that "legacy is the lasting impact of your life" (Legacy Project, 2021). Legacy is more than your life. Legacy encompasses prior generations, family stories, traditions, your heritage, as well as that which you leave for future generations. Whitman provides

DOI: 10.4324/9781003298168-2

an eloquent definition: "We go back to find the security of home, but also to find in the past the answer to the present" (1986, p. 121).

Ancestry claims genealogy, searching for one's roots, is the second most popular hobby in the United States (Dalzell, 2017). Genealogy was first used by the Europeans, who wanted to document their lineage for purposes of social standing or claims to inheritance as well as proving that they descended from royalty. European lineage can be traced back as early as 1300 and sometimes earlier. Dalzell (2017) contends that interest in learning about family history became popular in the United States in the 1960s. The digital era of the 1990s, when records became available online, resulted in a surge of activity as individuals did not have to travel to research facilities and repositories to view vital and historical records to conduct research. Interestingly, the first published work in the United States on genealogy was in 1771 (Genealogy Society of Utah, 1915).

Preserving One's Legacy

There are endless ways to explore and preserve one's legacy. Visiting places where your ancestors lived or are buried oftentimes proves to be a powerful experience in addition to acquiring a wealth of information. Ardis Whitman published an article in *Reader's Digest* in 1986 describing her pilgrimage with her granddaughter to Nova Scotia to visit Ardis's grandmother's home. This pilgrimage was both healing and meaningful. As she stood on the exact spot where her grandmother's house once stood, she recalled sweet times with her grandmother when she was young. Ardis tells the reader about these powerful childhood memories that helped her navigate difficult times throughout her life. She leaves us with the message, "[T]o know where I come from is one of the great longings of the heart" (Whitman, 1986, p. 119).

Writing a memoir, whether to self-publish to share with extended family or published works intended for a wider audience, provides lasting memories and life lessons for readers. There are countless authors who have written a memoir aimed to heal their past. These stories are therapeutic on multiple levels. A great example of healing is Cheryl Strayed's memoir, *Wild*. After losing her mother to a long battle with cancer and then divorcing her husband, Strayed (2012) follows her desire to travel and find the person she used to be. She shares with us her healing journey as she hikes the Pacific Crest Trail in California. This story is a great example of using the present to heal her past, which frees her to move into the future. Memoirs facilitate healing experiences for readers as their issues and themes connect with the author's challenges and healing journey. Appendix I contains a list of inspirational memoirs with brief descriptions. Reading meaning-filled memoirs helps foster a connection with, and memory of, one's emotional history.

Creating a family cookbook is a popular way to document and share family traditions. So many families have traditional foods handed down over many generations. Compiling a family cookbook involves connecting with relatives to obtain recipes and stories. Having various family members contribute recipes and the stories behind each recipe can be done in writing or submitted using an audio device oftentimes makes the process less daunting. There are software programs to help organize a family cookbook as well as numerous self-publishing options for making print copies and/or digital copies to share with the extended family. A family cookbook is a wonderful way to preserve the past and leave a legacy for future generations.

Another popular method for preserving one's legacy is by creating oral histories. It is easy to interview a family member using a smartphone or audio recording device to collect stories and be able to share them. One can also participate in large-scale oral history projects. Two examples are the Worcester Women's *Oral History Project*, which records and shares the personal histories of women from the Worcester, Massachusetts, area, and the *Veterans History Project*, where the US federal government collects and preserves written, audio and/or video recordings of veterans' stories. Several compelling works demonstrate that telling a family story contributes to a sense of community and can enhance one's identity and feelings of connectedness (Hadis, 2002; Merrill & Fivush, 2016). Please see Appendix II, as it provides a list of legacy projects for facilitators and group members to stimulate legacy exploration and preservation.

Purpose of Legacy Groups

The Legacy Model (Figure 1.1) provides a novel and innovative group experience and is developed to enhance wellness in adults. This therapeutic intervention is designed to promote psychological health through the healing power of legacy in a group setting. Group members engage in self-reflection and explore, preserve, and redefine for themselves their family history and traditions. Group members experience enhanced protective factors associated with psychological well-being. The Legacy Model components include engaging in self-reflection, exploring family history and traditions, deepening a sense of purpose in life, discovering one's roots, facilitating meaning-making, and preserving family legacy for future generations. Self-reflection exercises encourage group members to become aware of their thoughts, feelings, and family relationships while they explore some aspects of their ancestral legacy. Some individuals have the desire to create an artifact for future generations. Other members may want to learn about their ancestors, who they were, where they came from, what they did for work, their culture and stories of courage and hardship. Group facilitators encourage meaning-making and assist members in deepening their purpose in life.

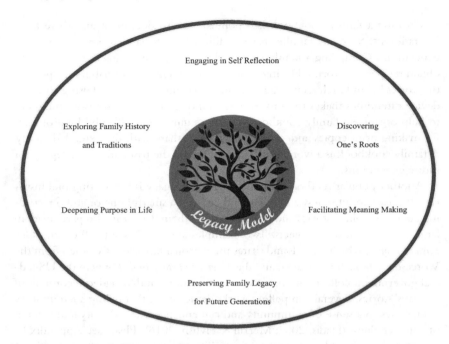

FIGURE 1.1 The components of the Legacy Model.

Merlino (2008) wrote about the benefits of researching family history. She identified six key benefits experienced by adults: a clear sense of purpose, enhanced identity, connection with living relatives and ancestors, cognitive stimulation, social interaction, and medical knowledge. Additional benefits for older adults have been noted by Weithers (2017) from the *We Have Kids* initiative. She contends that older adults show enhanced overall well-being, more specifically, feeling accomplished being able to research and compile their family history. Adults also show an increase in self-worth, as well as a sense of belonging to a larger ancestral community. Moore et al. (2021) contend that conducting genealogy is an altruistic activity as the researcher is leaving their legacy to future generations.

Genealogical research as a counseling intervention has shown great promise with different age groups. In 1985, Grace Paul wrote about her experience as a retired government worker who became a volunteer, helping nursing home residents research their family history and guiding them in sharing this information with younger family members. Some of the residents went on to publish articles. Paul (1985) observed a significant increase in energy when older adults thought about helping others. Erikson et al. (1994) contend that during this psychosocial stage of generativity, individuals show concern for the next generation. Champagne (1990) reported using genealogical searches as a counseling technique, exploring legacy with clients to enhance healing and personal growth. More recently, Foor (2017) published *Ancestral Medicine*, providing exercises and guidance for psychotherapists to work with clients by using their ancestral legacy work for health and healing. The book is a compilation of Foor's (2017) 20 years' experience observing the benefits with clients that include an increased sense of purpose and meaning-making.

The International Council on Active Aging was established in 2001 to foster wellness initiatives for older adults with the goal to "develop a culture of wellness" (ICAA, 2019). The ICAA Forum 2019 created a definition of wellness to share with all cultures across the world; "[W]ellness is derived from our ability to understand, accept and act upon our capacity to lead a purpose-filled and engaged life" (ICCA, 2019).

In keeping with the ICCA mission, the Legacy Model was designed to provide the practitioners with a guided process to enhance psychological wellness by exploring one's legacy and creating legacy projects. These projects draw upon family stories, traditions, and one's heritage to preserve these experiences for future generations. The Legacy Model is a novel and innovative approach that can be used as a counseling intervention to enhance self-reflection by exploring and preserving one's legacy.

References

Bosak, S. V. (2021). *Legacy project.* www.legacyproject.org

Champagne, D. E. (1990, October). The genealogical search as a counseling technique. *Journal of Counseling & Development, 69*(1), 85–87.

Dalzell, R. (2017, April). *Most popular hobby in the US?* http://Ancestry.blogs.ancestry. com/cm/genealogy-second-most-popular-hobby-us/

Erikson, E. H., Erikson, J. M., & Kivnick, H. Q. (1994). *Vital involvement in old age: The experience of old age in our times.* W.W. Norton & Company.

Foor, D. (2017). *Ancestral medicine: Rituals for personal and family healing.* Bear & Company.

Genealogy Society of Utah. (1915). *Lessons in genealogy.* https://openlibrary.org/books/ OL25401676M/Lessons_in_genealogy

Hadis, M. (2002). *From generation to generation: Family stories, computers and genealogy* [Master of Science in Media Technology thesis, Media Arts and Sciences, Massachusetts Institute of Technology]. www.dspace.mit.edu/handle/1721.1/61544

International Council on Active Aging Forum 2019. (2019). www.ICAA.cc//business/ wellness-model-htm

Legacy Project. (2021). *Legacy links.* www.legacyproject.org/7gen/legacylinks.html

Merlino, A. (2008, April). *Six surprising benefits of researching your family history.* www. czepigalaw.com/blog/6-surprising-benefits-of-researching-your-family-history/

Merrill, M., & Fivush, R. (2016). Intergenerational narratives and identity across development. *Developmental Review, 40*, 72–92.

Moore, S., Rosenthal, D., & Robinson, R. (2021). *The psychology of family history: Exploring our genealogy*. Routledge, Taylor & Francis Group.

Mouillot, M. R. (2015). *A fifty-year silence: Love, war, and a ruined house in France*. Crown Publishers.

Paul, G. (1985, June). Working on family trees: A form of resident therapy. *Nursing Homes, 34*(3), 41–42.

Strayed, C. (2012). *Wild*. Atlantic Books.

Weithers, D. (2017). *How older people benefit from knowing their genealogy*. www.wehavekids. com/family-relationships/How-Genealogy-Affects-Wellbeing-in-Older-People/

Whitman, A. (1986, April). You must go home again. *Readers Digest, 128*, 117–120.

2
THEORETICAL FRAMEWORK FOR THE LEGACY MODEL

The Legacy Model is a group intervention designed to promote psychological health through the healing power of legacy. Group members engage in self-reflection, explore some facet of their legacy, and redefine the meaning of their family history and traditions, with the goal of enhancing their psychological well-being. The Model is grounded in various existing and overlapping concepts and theories from the professional literature as no single theory or concept defines the processes of this innovative wellness group.

Aging and Development

According to US Census data (2020), there were 54.1 million adults aged 65 years and older in the United States in 2019. This accounts for 16 percent of the total US population. Population estimates for adults aged 65 years and older will reach 94.7 million by 2060 (Vespa et al., 2020), which reflects nearly one in four persons of the total US population will fall into this group. Medical advances have accounted for some of this growth as well as the explosive "Baby Boom" years that occurred between 1946 and 1964. Many of these "Boomers" are now reaching mid to late adulthood and find themselves reflecting on their lives and their legacy.

An important task of adulthood is the integration of psycho-socio-emotional and spiritual factors, which some theorists describe as developing a deeper under-standing of the self. Rohr (2011) contends that central to identity development in adulthood is "a desire for rediscovery of one's roots, one's traditions, one's symbols, one's ethnic identity, and one's own unique identity" (pp. 39–40). This continued growth is essential for building greater ego strength, a critical

DOI: 10.4324/9781003298168-3

component of resiliency as it enhances one's ability to cope with life stressors and contributes to overall psychological well-being.

Erikson (1980) contends that when adults reach midlife, they are met with the task of fostering and nurturing others and giving back to the world. Adults successfully move into "generativity" by raising children, mentoring younger persons, or possibly volunteering. According to Erikson, some adults may feel disconnected to their family or uninvolved in their community. As such, this can lead to stagnation. Older adulthood (aged >60 years) is a time for reflection on past accomplishments, roads taken, and a move toward building a sense of integrity. This is a time of self-reflection or what is referred to as life review. The Legacy Model draws from Erikson's psychosocial theory of development as well as the work of Vaillant (1993), who built upon Erikson's (1980) theory of development. According to Vaillant, for adults aged 60–75 years is a time for passing on knowledge and their cultural norms to future generations, that is, being keeper of the meaning. The reflective capabilities of this age group enable them to contemplate their place in the world often with the wisdom that Erikson (1980) first described. Vaillant (2012) suggests that successful aging leads to the acquisition of a sense of justice. Therefore, the gift of older adulthood lies in the potential to guide the next generation in a broader sense.

The ability to reflect on one's own experience while considering another person's place in the world is the first hint we are given at the concept of empathy and how this plays a role in successful aging. The Legacy Model is informed by this developmental perspective as the Legacy Group intervention was designed to foster and facilitate successful aging of the increasing population of older adults.

Foundational Group Work

The effectiveness and benefits of group counseling have been well documented over the past 30 years (Burlingame & Strauss, 2021). The Legacy Model uses a counseling group type as the focus is on personal growth (Association for Specialists in Group Work, 2021). The purpose of a Legacy Group is to assist the members in exploring their legacy and/or preserving a legacy project. Legacy Groups incorporate the therapeutic factors (Yalom & Leszcz, 2020), sometimes referred to as curative factors. These therapeutic factors are the cornerstones for therapeutic change and healing and serve as a therapeutic foundation for the Legacy Group curricula.

In reviewing the therapeutic factors, we know that establishing a safe and confidential group environment early fosters *group cohesion*, which is critical for a successful group experience. Sharing legacy experiences builds a sense of *universality* and most often leads to an *instillation of hope* for group members. Using various legacy exercises to stimulate members' awareness and help them get in touch with their life stories, memories, and ancestral legacy sets the stage for sharing and offering suggestions, *imparting of information*, to one another. It is customary for veterans and older adults to provide support and assistance generously, clearly a demonstration of *altruism*. A key role of the Legacy Group facilitator is to foster meaning-making with group members. This often invites *existential* queries as each member explores their legacy more deeply. Yalom and Leszcz (2020) contend that growth and change are linked to the therapeutic factors at play in the group process.

Rattenbury and Stone (1989) conducted research with nursing home residents who were assigned to one of the two group experiences: a reminiscence group or a current topics group. The researchers measured the psychological well-being pre- and post-group experience and included an index of individual participation levels during group time (i.e., talking score). The researchers reported that both groups, processing past experiences and current events, were strongly associated with gains in psychological well-being as measured by happiness and depression scales compared to residents who received no treatment intervention. Further, participation in group (i.e., talking score) was associated with psychological well-being improvement. Data collected on the Legacy Model similarly found that members experienced the healing power of group work. Other research suggests that incorporating tangibles (e.g., photographs, writing, audio recordings) into group work with older adults significantly enhances the group process and group outcomes (Christensen et al., 2006). As such, the Activity-Based Legacy Group curriculum was designed to incorporate the use of tangible artifacts with members.

James Birren focused his research on understanding and enhancing the psychological health of older adults for more than 40 years. Toward the end of his career, Birren developed *Guided Autobiography* (GAB) *Groups* (Birren & Cochran, 2001). These groups revolved around autobiography as "life stories, life review, reminiscences, memories, memoirs, and more" (p. 5). The purpose of the GAB intervention is to weave autobiography into a group experience with older adults. Results from GAB showed this group process had great therapeutic benefit for group members (Birren & Deutchman, 1991). Birren and Cochran (2001) reported measurable gains in emotional well-being for individuals who engaged in life review, which include the following (pp. 15–16):

- Increased self-esteem and a greater sense of personal power and significance.
- Greater awareness of past adaptive strategies and ways in which these might be applied to current problems and conditions.
- Resolution of past resentments, pain, and negative feelings and a sense of reconciliation.
- Renewed interests in past activities and hobbies.
- Ability to differentiate between the roles of enduring internal motivations and external societal motivations in making life choices.
- Development of friendships and confidant relationships with other group members.

- An increased sense of meaning in life.
- Appreciation for the developmental work one faces at each stage of life.
- A greater sense of accomplishment and fulfillment.
- A stronger, more positive view of the future.

Birren's own legacy can be found on The Birren Center for Autobiographical Studies website (https://guidedautobiography.com/), where the Center continues to provide training and collect data about the value of practitioner insight regarding healing long-standing emotional issues in ancestral legacy. More recent research suggests that individuals do not need to share a full or even lengthy autobiography to gain psychological benefit. Individuals finding joy and purpose in their career are more likely to experience aspects of psychological well-being (Rath & Harter, 2010). Therefore, groups that focus on applying meaning to one's work may be particularly beneficial.

Finding Meaning in Medicine (FFM) *Groups* (Remen, 2002) offer an opportunity for those in caregiving fields to share their at-work experiences with their peers who get it. The experience of sharing stories as well as listening to others reportedly increases job satisfaction and minimizes burnout. Groups are self-led or co-facilitated by a physician and a mental health professional (Bertram, 2017). In either case, a topic or theme is presented for the session (i.e., healing, empathy, loss) and each member chooses to share or not. To keep the group on a personal note, members are asked to use "I" statements and avoid referring to the medical literature. As a result, members have reported feeling less isolated, less stressed, and more able to bring their own values and perspectives to the work of medicine (Remen, 2002). Further, renewed appreciation for the emotional rewards of the job and an overall increase in psychological well-being have been reported by Bertram (2017).

Like GAB and FFM, Narrative Therapy offers a platform in which clients tell and retell their stories. Narrative therapy involves assisting clients with exploring their beliefs, skills, behavior patterns, and, more significantly, the history of where and how these qualities arose. Clients may enter counseling for a variety of reasons; however, the therapist helps the client co-author a new narrative based on the truths, challenges, and desired changes that result from their exploration. In narrative therapy there is no one single truth or reality but only the many different interpretations we apply to our own reality and, more importantly, the meaning and power we ascribe to it. Narrative theorists suggest that all people create meaning through the stories they tell (i.e., narratives) about themselves. More significantly, individuals continue to live their lives according to those truths. A necessary component of change then is the understanding that there is no one knowable self but, instead, many selves, and a new self is just a story away (Hutto & Gallagher, 2017; Etchinson & Kleist, 2000).

Contributions of Intergenerational Theory

Intergenerational theory contends that our values, behaviors, family patterns, and actions (both positive and negative) are transmitted through ancestral lines (Jones, 2012). This transmission occurs via observable means such as passed down family traditions and communication styles, and through much less discernable paths as information is transferred energetically, neurobiologically, and even unconsciously from individual to individual, and from family to family through generations. This is observed as unfinished business that occurs in a family of origin and continues to impact future generations through passed down secrets and unspoken loyalties (Fishbane, 2016). Individuals that seek counseling for emotional or relationship issues may find liberation in the realization that their thought patterns and behaviors have been subtly normalized, even encouraged over many generations. However, others may not progress in psychotherapy as they may have difficulty letting go of blame, negative identification, and other forms of resistance that keep them locked in their story and their life narrative (Fishbane, 2016).

Bowen Family Systems and Contextual Therapy offer a slightly different perspective regarding intergenerational therapy. Both theories are rooted in the philosophy that people do not exist in a vacuum and their life experiences cannot be separated from their generational roots. Instead, therapy is focused on healthy differentiation. One way this focus is garnered is with the use of genograms – developed by Bowen (1980), an intergenerational family theorist – as a therapeutic tool in counseling since the 1980s (Magnuson & Shaw, 2003). Using a diagram to depict multigenerational family legacies allows therapists to identify emotional processes in the family that influence the functioning and health of individual family members.

In *Solving People Problems*, Sandwell (2008) explains how he uses genograms for assessment in psychotherapy by constructing a three to five generational family history with clients. Sandwell has found this to be effective in addressing emotional wounds and dysfunctional behaviors. His goal is to assist clients in looking as far back as needed to identify themes and patterns. Raising awareness is the first step to potentially improving the quality of current relationships and future generations. Another strategy employed by intergenerational therapists is to assist the client with waking from the spell of childhood (Fishbane, 2019). In doing so, clients may see their parents (or others) as real persons who experienced their own struggles, challenges, successes, and failures. In doing so, clients can make peace with aspects of their childhood and come to understand and even forgive their parents and themselves. With this process, individuals are empowered to take control of, and responsibility for, their life as they begin to move away from a hierarchical view toward a generational view of their parents and their legacy. Some clients will have the desire and opportunity to make changes in their relationships, perhaps for the first time, enjoying an adult-to-adult relationship with their parents, forever changing the future of their interactions (Fishbane, 2016).

Culture and Context: Intergenerational Theories

Let's Hold Hands and Drop Dead: Three Generations, One Story by Cooper (2015) is a cleverly articulated account of the author's personal reflections on childhood and the links she observed about her father's legacy while facilitating an adult therapy group. Cooper draws heavily from the work of Carl Jung that incorporates the social unconscious, also called the generational unconscious, which revolves around buried memories from past generational trauma. The traumatic events, she suggests, may have occurred one or two generations earlier, and the client is unaware of this trauma or its impact on their life. Historical and cultural traumas can have a very powerful negative impact on subsequent generations.

Deangelis (2019) reviewed several studies about the effects of trauma across generations and contends that not only is an individual affected but the traumatic experience ripples outward to adversely influence familial, social, and cultural systems. The trauma experienced may have a greater impact than first believed. Although the psychological effects of generational trauma on an individual have been widely accepted, Deangelis (2019) goes on to suggest that intergenerational-cultural trauma also induces change at the neurobiological and possibly even the genetic levels. Ongoing studies with Holocaust survivors and their descendants suggest atypically high rates of anxiety, depression, and post-traumatic stress disorder (Deangelis, 2019). Interestingly, Danieli (2016) suggests that the various adaptive and reparative behaviors among the descendants are generational in nature and help explain observed differences.

Similarly, the effects of intergenerational-cultural trauma have been observed among Native American descendants. One example is the Canadian government's attempts from the 1880s to the mid-1990s to eliminate the Indian problem. The education offered to Native American children during this time involved teaching children to be ashamed of their cultural heritage and traditions. As a result, children and grandchildren of the survivors have experienced an overall decrease in well-being, including emotional (i.e., psychological distress, suicide attempts), cognitive (i.e., learning disabilities), and physical (i.e., likelihood of contracting disease) (Bombay et al., 2014). This, and similar research (Hartmann et al., 2019) regarding racial and historical trauma, has led to the development of resilience-promoting interventions designed to heal intergenerational wounds (Fishbane, 2016).

Neurobiology Advances

Advances in neuroscience and technology have led to research investigations about the transferring of intergenerational information which may begin at the neurobiological level, particularly in the way we form memories and initial attachments. Siegel (2012) contends that memory is a catalyst for the way in which a past experience alters the probability of how the mind functions in the future and that the process of encoding information alters future ways of responding to other people and with one's environment. This broader conceptualization of memory opens the door for new considerations regarding the impact of life's earliest experiences.

Explicit memories are those that clients can draw upon consciously and intentionally. They are memories involving facts (i.e., semantic memory) and events (i.e., episodic memory). It is the combination of these aspects of explicit memory that helps us place our self in time and forms a narrative to tell our life story. Significantly, when clients utilize explicit memory, there is an internal experience of remembering; however, this is not the case with implicit memory. Implicit memories are unconscious. They are triggered by interactions with the present environment and without the internal sensation of remembering. Clients may report being overwhelmed by feelings that seemingly come from nowhere. This cycle of feeling–thought–behavior is the result of a neuronal stimulation deeply rooted in their neurobiology (Fishbane, 2005; Siegel, 2012). To form explicit memory, the hippocampus must be utilized, yet this brain region is not formed until approximately 18 months of age. Infants then (<18 months) rely on the perceptual and somatosensory information that is encoded in the limbic system and available at birth to form implicit memory. This same emotional brain is responsible in part for the initial attachments (i.e., feeling secure, anxious, disorganized) that are so critical for future relationship processing (Fishbane, 2005; Siegel, 2012). Schemas, or mental representations, are created for all aspects of our world, and as research suggests, that once formed it is in our nature to seek out familiar patterns that match our existing schemas (Siegel, 2012). It has been shown that we are "wired for habit" neurologically: the more one does, feels, or thinks something, the more likely one is to do, feel, or think the same again. Those neural paths are strengthened with each traverse. Or as Hebb first suggested as early as 1949: neurons that fire together, wire together (Fishbane, 2005; Hebb, 2002; Siegel, 2012). Fortunately, in the same way that we are wired for familiarity, research suggests that we are also wired for change.

Fishbane (2019) states that our brain is capable of change throughout the lifespan, not only creating new connections between neurons (i.e., neuroplasticity) but also generating new neurons (i.e., neurogenesis). Counseling that involves this type of neuropsycho-education is beneficial, in that clients become aware of how individual and familial habits are formed in the brain and what strategies and challenges are involved in breaking them. Older adults benefit from neuropsycho-education; while engaging in certain tasks, they incorporate more of both brain hemispheres than younger clients. As a result, there is an increase in the integration of experiences that leads to a broadening of perspective-taking, a greater flexibility of thought, and an increase in resilience and wisdom (Fishbane, 2005). Both the Process-Focused Legacy Groups (Chapter 5) and the Activity-Based Legacy Groups (Chapter 6) draw upon these neurobiological advances to inform legacy activities used in the group experience.

Psychological Well-Being

Like many constructs in social science, defining a term can be challenging; psychological well-being proves no different. As early as 1969, the Bradburn Model suggested that psychological well-being was associated with having a positive attitude (Bradburn, 1969). Over time, definitions of psychological well-being have expanded and grown more in depth. A widely used definition from the Foresight Project team on Mental Capital and Wellbeing defined mental well-being as "a dynamic state, in which the individual is able to develop their potential, work productively and creatively, build strong and positive relationships with others and contribute to their community" (Beddington et al., 2008, p. 1057). This definition was adopted and served to inform the development of the Legacy Model.

The Legacy Model was developed for veterans and older adults. Evidence-based research on these two populations suggest strong associations between stress and a decline in health and well-being, including mental, emotional, and behavioral disorders, which are thought to be preventable as documented by the National Research Council and Institute of Medicine (2009). Given this, the World Health Organization (2018) stated that promoting mental health and emotional well-being is central to successful aging. Similarly, Mental Health America (2016) *Position Statement 35* advocates for strategies and interventions aimed at enhancing mental health and wellness with the intention of improving quality of life and reducing healthcare costs. Research consistently shows that psychosocial interventions (i.e., support groups, psychoeducation) increase wellness and quality of life, whereas no drug demonstrates the same effectiveness (Australian Psychological Society, 2018).

The US Department of Veterans Affairs (2020) data show that there were 19,541,961 veterans in the United States in 2020. The National Council for Behavioral Health (2019) report that less than 50 percent of military returning from overseas received treatment for mental health concerns and that approximately 22 veterans die by suicide every day. The Center for New American Security funded a research to define wellness and recommended holistic treatment options for veterans. This research resulted in the report, *Well after Service* (Berglass & Harrell, 2012), that strongly recommends achieving wellness beyond symptom reduction. The *Veterans Wellness Model* (Berglass & Harrell, 2012) was created to provide guidance, with efforts to achieve physical and psychological well-being for veterans by integrating four domains of well-being, including purpose, material needs, health, and social/personal relationships. Three of these domains, purpose, health, and social/personal relationships, have been incorporated into the Legacy Model.

Exploring Ancestral Legacy

Psychological well-being efforts include healing wounds and broken relationships. Exploring one's ancestral legacy as a counseling strategy has shown to enhance an individual's mental health (Chance, 1988). DeSalvo (1999) contends that writing our stories can be transformative, resulting in an increased global understanding that improves our connection with our children, extended family, and with the environment. Exploring legacy provides the vehicle to no longer just view the past but, instead, act as an agency, as such, one can actively preserve it: family stories, values, traditions, and wisdom (Champagne, 1990; Grosskopf, 1999; Taylor, 2011).

A two-part process, exploring and preserving, appears to be the key for facilitating and fostering psychological wellness. Adopted children often engage in a quest to feel connected with their family of origin while also enhancing the relationships with their adoptive families (Triseliotis, 1998). Life Story Theory of Identity (Hunter & Rowles, 2005) offers a multifaceted and complex understanding as to why adopted children, as well as others, engage in legacy exploration and preservation. Individuals find ways of grounding themselves in their past and in their future, allowing themselves to move beyond generational thinking and into legacy thinking (Hunter & Rowles, 2005), and form healthy family identities (Reiser, 2012). Family stories become more important than family things, as individuals engaged in this process report an increased sense of gratification, satisfaction, accomplishment, and improved self-esteem (Unfleet, 2009).

Key aspects of each of the highlighted concepts and theories have been interwoven to inform the Legacy Model (see Figure 2.1). First, we recognize the need for a safe and supportive space in which the transformative power of the therapeutic factors group process occurs. Second, we acknowledge the significance of legacy stories created as they relate to the past, the present, and the future. Further, there is the belief that changes in one individual can be transformative for the entire family system, in the present and for generations to come. The relational-neurobiological approach suggests that ancestral wisdom may be used to understand, contextualize, and empathize with one's legacy and can potentially be a healing process (Fishbane, 2016). Awareness of challenges in the family of origin often initiates making meaning of, and a desire to pass along, a healthy emotional legacy that can become a key motivator for change (Macleod et al., 2014). Empathy toward present and past (i.e., self and parents) is an important component to stimulate true healing. Legacy Groups offer a safe and supportive space for group members to embark on this journey.

The Legacy Model is grounded in the notion that psychological health and well-being is enhanced when an individual is given the opportunity to feel empowered through the exploration and meaning-making process. This is one of the primary benefits of the Model, as the Legacy Group curricula were designed to promote wellness using a group prevention practice that increases connection with the family, improves social supports, and offers a safe environment to explore and clarify the meaning of their life. Further, engaging in legacy exploration and preservation enhances protective factors while simultaneously reducing risk factors, thereby increasing overall psychological well-being. The Legacy Model is

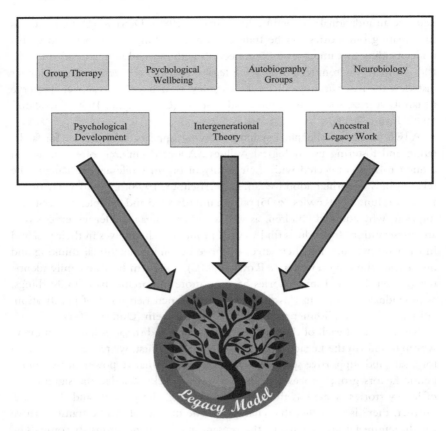

FIGURE 2.1 The Legacy Model. The theories that informed the Legacy Model.

grounded in the theoretical framework described that is related to self, family, community, and globally. We can all benefit from drawing connections, seeking answers to questions, and sometimes letting go of the perceptually unchangeable past to heal the future.

References

Association for Specialists in Group Work. (2021). *ASGW guiding principles for group work.* https://asgw.org/wp-content/uploads/2021/07/ASGW-Guiding-Principles-May-2021.pdf

Australian Psychological Society. (2018). *Evidenced-based psychological interventions in the treatment of mental disorders: A review of the literature* (4th ed.). https://psychology.org.au/getmedia/23c6a11b-2600-4e19-9a1d-6ff9c2f26fae/evidence-based-psych-interventions.pdf

Beddington, J., Cooper, C. L., Field, J., Goswami, U., Huppert, F. A., Jenkins, R., Johns, H. S., Kirkwood, B. L., Sahakian, B. J., & Thomas, S. M. (2008). The mental wealth of nations. *Nature, 455*(23), 1057–1060. www.mentalhealthpromotion.net/resources/mental_wealth_nations_nature.pdf

Berglass, N. & Harrell, M. C. (2012). *Well after service: Veteran reintegration and American communities.* Center for New American Security.

Bertram, B. (2017). Story-telling: Finding meaning in work. *The Group Worker, 46*(1), 9–11.

Birren, J. E., & Cochran, K. N. (2001). *Telling the stories of life through guided autobiography groups.* Johns Hopkins University Press.

Birren, J. E., & Deutchman, D. E. (1991). *Guiding autobiography groups for older adults.* Johns Hopkins University Press.

Bombay, A., Matheson, K., & Anison, H. (2014). The intergenerational effects of Indian residential schools: Implications for the concept of historical trauma. *Transcultural Psychiatry, 51*(3), 320–338.

Bowen, M. (1980). *Key to the genogram.* Georgetown University Hospital.

Bradburn, N. M. (1969). *The structure of psychological well-being.* Aldine.

Burlingame, G. M., & Strauss, B. (2021). Efficacy of small group treatments: Foundation for evidence-based practice. In M. Barkham, W. Lutz, & L. G. Castonguay (Eds.), *Bergin and Garfield's handbook of psychotherapy and behavior change* (7th ed., p. 119). John Wiley & Sons, Inc.

Champagne, D. E. (1990). The genealogical search as a counseling technique. *Journal of Counseling and Development, 69*, 85–87.

Chance, S. (1988). The psychological functions of genealogy in the aged. *Journal of Geriatric Psychiatry and Neurology, 1*, 113–115.

Christensen, T. M., Hulse-Killacky, D., Salgado, R. A., Thornton, M. D., & Miller, J. L. (2006). Facilitating reminiscence groups: Perceptions of group leaders. *Journal of Specialist in Group Work, 31*(1), 73–88.

Cooper, E. J. (2015). *Let's hold hands and drop dead: Three generations, one story.* Morgan James Publishing.

Danieli, Y. (2016). Group project for Holocaust survivors and their children. *American Journal of Orthopsychiatry, 86*(6), 639–651.

Deangelis, T. (2019, February). Legacy of trauma. *Monitor on Psychology, 50*(2), 36.

DeSalvo, L. (1999). *Writing as a way of healing: How telling our stories transforms our lives.* Harper.

Erikson, E. (1980). *Identity and the life cycle.* W.W. Norton & Company.

Etchinson, M., & Kleist, D. M. (2000). Review of narrative therapy: Research and utility. *The Family Journal: Counseling and Therapy for Couples and Families, 8*(1), 61–66.

Fishbane, M. D. (2005). Differentiation and dialogue in intergenerational relationships. In J. Lebow (Ed.), *Handbook of clinical family therapy* (pp. 543–568). John Wiley.

Fishbane, M. D. (2016). The neurobiology of relationships. In T. L. Sexton & J. Lebow (Eds.), *Handbook of family therapy* (pp. 48–65). Routledge, Taylor & Francis Group.

Fishbane, M. D. (2019, December). Healing intergenerational wounds: An integrative relational-neurobiological approach. *Family Process, 58*(4), 796–818.

Grosskopf, B. (1999). *Forgive your parents, heal yourself: How understanding your painful family legacy can transform your life.* The Free Press.

Hartmann, W. E., Wendt, D. C., Burrage, R. L., Pomerville, A., & Gone, J. P. (2019). American Indian historical trauma: Anticolonial prescriptions for healing, resilience, and survivance. *American Psychologist, 74*(1), 6–19.

Hebb, D. O. (2002). *The organization of behavior: A neuropsychological theory.* Taylor & Francis eLibrary, 2009.

Hunter, E. G., & Rowles, G. D. (2005). Leaving a legacy: Toward a typology. *Journal of Aging Studies, 19*(3), 327–347.

Hutto, D. D., & Gallagher, S. (2017). Re-authoring narrative therapy: Improving our self-management tools. *Philosophy, Psychiatry and Psychology, 24*(2), 157–167.

Jones, S. (2012, October 25–28). *The dynamics of intergenerational behavior and forgiveness therapy* [Paper presentation]. North American of Christians in Social Work Convention. www.nacsw.org/Publications/Proceedings2012/JonesSTheDynamicsFINAL.pdf

Macleod, D. J., Sadewa, A. B., Arthur, R. A., Collins, K. L., Hand-Breckenridge, T. L., Runstedler, Y., & Van Hooren, K. A. (2014). The balance of fairness in family relations: A contextual family therapy case study. *Consensus, 35*(2), Article 6. http://scholars.wlu.ca/consensus/vol35/iss2/6

Magnuson, S., & Shaw, S. (2003). Adaptations of the multifaceted genogram in counseling, training, and supervision. *The Family Journal, 11*(1), 45–54.

Mental Health America. (2016). *Position statement 35: Aging well: Wellness and psychological treatment for the emotional and cognitive challenges of aging.* http//www.mentalhealth-america.net/positions/aging-well

National Council for Behavioral Health. (2019). *Veterans.* www.thenationalcouncil.org/topics/veterans/

National Research Council (US) and Institute of Medicine (US). (2009). Committee on the prevention of mental disorders and substance abuse among children, youth, and young adults: Research advances and promising interventions. In M. E. O'Connell, T. Boat, & K. E. Warner (Eds.), *Preventing mental, emotional, and behavioral disorders among young people: Progress and possibilities.* National Academies Press. www.ncbi.nlm.nih.gov/books/NBK32775/

Rath, T., & Harter, J. (2010). *Wellbeing: The essential elements.* Gallup, Inc.

Rattenbury, C., & Stones, M. J. (1989, December). A controlled evaluation of reminiscence and current topics discussion groups in nursing home context. *Gerontologist, 29*(6), 768–771.

Reiser, M. L. (2012). *Exploring genealogical roots and family history and their influence on college student development: A qualitative study* [Theses and Dissertations, Brigham Young University]. Paper 3356.

Remen, R. N. (2002). *Finding meaning in medicine: Forming an FMM conversation group. A resource guide for medical students.* Institute for the Study of Health and Wellness, A Commonwealth Project. https://rishiprograms.org/wp-content/uploads/FMMStu-dentResourceGuide.pdf

Rohr, R. (2011). *Falling upward.* Jossey-Bass.

Sandwell, P. G. (2008). *Solving people problems for the creation and preservation of family wealth.* Salt Pond Press.

Siegel, D. J. (2012). *The developing mind: How relationships and the brain interact to shape who we are* (2nd ed.). Guilford Press.

Taylor, D. (2011). *Creating a spiritual legacy: Passing on your stories, values, and wisdom.* Brajos Press.

Triseliotis, J. (1998). Identify and genealogy in adopted people. In D. Brodjinsky (Ed)., *Children's adjustment to adoption: Developmental and clinical issues* (pp. 35–43). Sage Publications.

Unfleet, S. B. (2009). *Genealogy and generativity in older adults* [Theses and Dissertations,. San Jose State University].

United States Census Bureau. (2020). *The population 65 years and older in the United States: 2019.* www.census.gov/topics/population/older-aging.html

United States Department of Veterans Affairs. (2020). www.va.gov/vetdata/docs/Quickfacts/stats_at_a_glance_6_30_21pdf

Vaillant, G. E. (1993). *The wisdom of the ego.* Harvard University Press.

Vaillant, G. E. (2012). Positive mental health: Is there a cross-cultural definition? *World Psychiatry, 11*(2), 93–99.

Vespa, J., Medina, L., & Armstrong, D. M. (2020). *Demographic turning points for the United States: Population projections for 2020 to 2060.* US Census Bureau. www.census.gov/content/dam/Census/library/publications/2020/demo/p25-1144.pdf

World Health Organization. (2018). *Mental health: Strengthening our response.* www.who.int/news-room/fact-sheets/detail/mental-health-strengthening-our-response

Yalom, I. D., & Leszcz, M. (2020). *The theory and practice of group psychotherapy* (6th ed.). Basic Books.

3
MEASURING THE EFFECTIVENESS OF THE LEGACY MODEL

This chapter provides information about the multiyear research study, wellness instrument used, the procedure, data collected from 2013 to 2019, and research study findings. Foremost in the foundation of this community service program and research study is the mission of the Legacy Group project (Box 3.1).

BOX 3.1   THE MISSION OF LEGACY GROUPS

The mission of the Legacy Group Project is to offer Legacy Groups to community members, which provide an opportunity for individuals to explore and preserve their legacy: that is, gain knowledge and meaning that enhance psychological wellness and connection as a global citizen. The Legacy Group Project aims to connect generations with their heritage by engaging in the exploration and preservation of their legacy, which provides a vehicle for sharing wisdom, values, and life experiences that reflects on and understands the past; engages and educates the present; and concretely preserves and guides future generations on their family history.

The idea for developing a Legacy Group intervention had been percolating since 1996. The Group Model was developed in 2011, followed by the delivery of a community service and research project that began in 2012, with grant funding for a pilot program to conduct Legacy Groups with women veterans. See Table 3.1 for a brief review of the process that guided the research team during this multiyear project.

DOI: 10.4324/9781003298168-4

TABLE 3.1 Overview of Multiyear Project: Conducting Groups and Collecting Data

Academic Year	Project Goals	Resources and Project Objectives
2012–2013	Idea Development and Resource Requests	• Bridgewater State University's (BSU's) Commitment of Resources • Legacy Group Team Formed • Created the Process-Focused Legacy Group Curriculum
2013–2014	Pilot Program Implemented with Data Collection	• Daughters of the American Revolution (DAR) Special Projects Grant with BSU Matching Funds and Research Assistant • Conducted Legacy Group with Women Veterans

2014–2015	Full Project Implementation with Data Collection	• BSU Presidential Fellowship
		• Conducted Legacy Groups with
		  • Veterans and Affiliates of Veterans and
		  • Older Adults

2015–2016	Full Project Implementation with Data Collection	• Post Fellowship Funds Expended
		• Conducted Legacy Groups with
		  • Veterans and Affiliates of Veterans and
		  • Older Adults
		• Community Settings
		• Assisted Living
		• Skilled Nursing Care
		• Created Activity-Based Legacy Curriculum

2016–2017	Full Project Implementation with Data Collection	• BSU Research Grant Award
		• Conducted Legacy Groups with
		  • Veterans and Affiliates of Veterans and
		  • Older Adults
		• Community Settings
		• Assisted Living
		• Skilled Nursing Care

2017–2018	Full Project Implementation with Data Collection	• Rotary Club of the Bridgewater Grant
		• Conducted Legacy Groups with
		  • Veterans and Affiliates of Veterans and
		  • Older Adults
		• Community Settings
		• Assisted Living
		• Skilled Nursing Care

(*Continued*)

TABLE 3.1 (Continued)

Academic Year	Project Goals	Resources and Project Objectives

2018–2019	Full Project Implementation with Data Collection and Data Analysis	• Rotary Club of the Bridgewater Grant
		• Conducted Legacy Groups with
		  • Veterans and Affiliates of Veterans and
		  • Older Adults
		• Community Settings
		• Assisted Living
		• Skilled Nursing Care

Measuring the Effectives of an Intervention

Evidence-based practice interventions are central to the delivery of mental health care in the United States. The American Psychological Association Guidelines (2021) state: "Psychologists strive to promote overall patient health, functioning, and well-being" (p. 18). There are several ways to measure the effectiveness of an intervention, which include using clinical judgment, reviewing the literature, and conducting quality research (American Group Psychotherapy Association, 2015; APA Presidential Task Force on Evidenced-Based Practice, 2006). The research team used guidelines recommended by the Presidential Task Force on Evidenced-Based Practice (2006) that have been implemented and utilized by the medical field in the United States for over 20 years. Effectiveness is measured by assessing two overarching client–outcome criteria: treatment efficacy (i.e., does the treatment work) and clinical utility (i.e., how relevant, and accessible is it).

The Theoretical Framework for the Legacy Model (Chapter 2) provides an overview of theories and concepts, as well as the underpinnings of ancestral legacy, which have been shown to be beneficial for enhancing psychological health, as such, informed the development of the Legacy Group intervention. The exploration of one's ancestry serves as a healing source for some individuals, while the preservation of that legacy offers a mechanism to share experiences and wisdom with future generations (i.e., generativity).

Legacy Groups were conducted as a no-cost, community-based group intervention. Legacy Team members reached out to community programs and directors, supplied flyers to academic and clinical programs, and created a website to reach out to potential group members about this opportunity. The groups were offered on a variety of days/times and in a variety of settings to ensure accessibility for potential members.

Enhancing Wellness with the Legacy Group Intervention

Life challenges and stressors associated with being a veteran and/or older adult are linked to a decline in overall health and wellness (APA, 2019; Bergeron & Smith, 2018). Psychological well-being is a global priority, as healthy people contribute to healthy communities and reduce the burden of disease on national budgets (US Department of Health & Human Services, 2022).

The Legacy Model is designed to promote psychological wellness using a group intervention designed to increase an individual's connection with self and family. It was hypothesized that adults who engage in a Legacy Group will experience improved psychological well-being, as measured by an increase in one or more constructs of the Ryff Scale of Psychological Well-Being (Ryff, 2014). Utilizing the theoretical concepts and instrumentation described, the research study questions were as follows:

1. How does overall psychological well-being change, based on the differences observed in pre-test and post-test scores?
2. How do pre-test scores differ from post-test scores based on gender, age, and member status?
3. How does psychological well-being change in each of the six constructs based on the differences observed in pre-test and post-test scores?
4. How do pre-test scores differ from post-test scores for each of the six constructs of psychological well-being based on gender, age, and member status?
5. How are pre-test and post-test scores different for individual items within each construct?
6. How are scores different for individual items based on gender, age, and member status?

Ryff Scales of Psychological Well-Being

The Ryff Scales of Psychological Well-Being (PWB) is a widely used instrument designed to measure psychological wellness (Ryff, 2014; Seifert, 2005). According to Ryff, previously available measures based loosely on theory and poorly defined terms and measures suggested that psychological wellness could be measured by an individual's score on an affect or life satisfaction scale. Ryff hypothesized that utilizing such broad measures resulted in skewed, value-laden criteria and a potential to neglect key features of wellness. Instead, she identified converging themes throughout the existing measures and attempted to integrate them into more clearly defined terms (Ryff, 2014, 1989).

Ryff (1989) identified six core constructs of psychological well-being, including Self-acceptance (SA), personal relation with others (PRO), autonomy (AU), environmental mastery (EM), purpose in life (PL), and personal growth (PG) (Box 3.2). After a series of preliminary tests, Ryff identified a 20-question scale for each construct consisting of (10) positive and (10) negative questions. Item-to-scale correlations were strong ranging from 0.86 to 0.93. Test–retest coefficients were also strong, ranging from 0.81 to 0.88, both supporting a confidence in the reliability of the measure. Ryff (1989) further observed that each construct was positively correlated to previous measures of positive functioning ($r = 0.25 - 0.73$, $p < 0.001$) and negatively correlated to previous measures of negative functioning ($r = -0.30 - -0.60$, $p < 0.001$), offering evidence for the validity of the scale. Strong intercorrelations were observed between each scale ($r = 0.32 - 0.76$), suggesting that all constructs were related to one overarching theme (well-being); yet she was able to present evidence to support the discreteness of each variable as well. Further, three scales (PRO, AU, and PG) did not correlate well with previous measures used throughout the literature ($0.25 - 0.45$), suggesting that these constructs had not been represented well in the other wellness scales (Ryff, 1989).

BOX 3.2 CONSTRUCTS OF PWB

Self-Acceptance – a positive attitude toward one's current self as well as their past self.

Positive Relationship with Others – warm, trusting interpersonal relationships, including those involving intimacy. Capacity to give and receive love, empathy, and generativity.

Autonomy – self-determination and independence; regulate behavior from within (internal locus of control); and sense of freedom from norms of everyday life.

Environmental Mastery – proactive participation in activities outside the self; ability to physically and mentally create, choose, and manipulate one's environment.

Purpose in Life – malleable but consistent goals and intentions; direction and sense of meaning.

Personal Growth – an openness to change and a willingness to confront new challenges, ongoing development of true potential.

Source: Ryff, C. D. (2014). Psychological well-being revisited: Advances in the science and practice of eudaimonia. *Psychotherapy and Psychosomatics*, *83*, 10–28. doi:10.1159/000353263

Three versions of the Ryff Scales of Psychological Well-Being have been developed (Ryff, 1989). The longest version has 84 items; the shortest has nine items. The short version is not recommended for use due to poor validity scores. The 54-item Ryff scale was selected for this research study. This instrument is based on a participant's response to questions on a six-point Likert scale ranging from 1 (strongly disagree) to 6 (strongly agree). Subscales are weighted equally, with each consisting of nine items mixed in throughout the assessment. Approximately half the items are reverse-scored, and the total subscale scores range between 9 and 54 (Ryff, 1989). In 2013, Dr. Carol Ryff generously supplied the instrument, scoring information, and 21 pages referencing research studies using the Ryff Scales of Psychological Well-Being for use in this research study.

Sample Selection

Participants were recruited for Legacy Groups, using flyers distributed to veteran groups and to organizations serving older adults in Southeastern Massachusetts. Direct outreach to program administrators of various organizations proved beneficial in reaching potential research study participants. During the pilot program year (2013–2014), Legacy Groups were conducted among women veterans, in keeping with grant-funding guidelines. In 2014, participation was broadened to include all older adults, aged 55–100 plus years. Legacy Groups were conducted from 2013 to 2019 and were approved by the Institutional Review Board for Research with Human Subjects at the university where the research project was conducted. Interested individuals attended informational sessions, completed a screening questionnaire, and received a copy of the *Call for Volunteers*, which provided detailed information about what to expect from the Legacy Group experience. In addition, all participants were given an informed consent form with an explanation of the process and instrument used in this study (e.g., Ryff Scales of Psychological Well-Being). Participation was voluntary. As such, participants could decline to complete the pre- and post-tests and continue attending the group experience or terminate at any time.

During informational sessions, interested individuals were invited to share their interest and readiness to explore their family legacy. The concept, keeper of the meaning (Vaillant, 1993), was shared with individuals and how meaning-making about individual legacies might look like in the group experience. Exclusion criteria consisted of persons with medical or psychiatric conditions that were not deemed a good fit for the Legacy Group experience.

Legacy Groups were conducted, and pre- and post-data were collected over seven years (2013–2019). Fifty participants completed a Legacy Group experience and the pre-post instrument. Each group was facilitated with two mental health professionals. Twelve Legacy Groups were conducted over the seven-year period, each group consisting of three to eight members. All Legacy Groups met for 12 hours consisting of 8–10 sessions. The length of the sessions varied, depending upon the unique needs of the group members. Process-Focused Legacy Groups (see Chapter 5) typically ran for 90 minutes, whereas Activity-Based Legacy Groups (see Chapter 6) conducted in long-term care facilities met for 45–60 minutes, as recommended by the hosting professional staff. All group members completed the Ryff scales during the first Legacy Group session. After the completion of the group experience, the Ryff instrument was mailed to group members one or two weeks later.

Baseline Characteristics

The research study sample consisted of 50 participants (N = 50); the average age of participants was 70.2 years (Standard Deviation (SD) = 14.3). Most participants were female (83.7 percent) and reported non-veteran status (77.6 percent). Seven participants did not complete either a pre- or a post-test, 20 completed only a pre-test, and one completed only a post-test. These participants were dropped from the analysis, resulting in 22 matched pairs. As seen in Table 3.2, the participants in the analysis sample (N = 22) were younger than the original sample, with an average age of 66 years (SD = 13.4); primarily female (90.9 percent), with a greater percentage of veterans than the initial sample (31.8 percent). Of the analyzed data set, "Affiliated" participants are those who reported associations with veterans or those in active duty (36.4 percent) and "general members" are those reporting non-veteran and no affiliation with veterans or others in active duty (31.8 percent). Twenty individual test items were missing (3 pre-test; 17 post-test). The items were imputed based on rounding sample means for each test item. For example, if the Test Number mean was 4.05, the input number was rounded to 4. If the Test Number was 1.95, the input number was rounded to 2. The result was a final sample of 22 completed pre- and post-tests.

Baseline associations between constructs are displayed in Table 3.3. As explained by Ryff (1989), each of the variables measured an aspect of a larger concept, well-being, so positive correlations are expected. EM was strongly associated with four other constructs (SA = 0.78, $p < 0.01$; PG = 0.72, $p < 0.01$; PL = 0.65, $p < 0.01$; PRO = 0.64, $p < 0.01$) and moderately associated with one (AU = 0.44, $p < 0.01$). PG was strongly associated with three constructs (EM = 0.72, $p < 0.01$; PL = 0.64, $p < 0.01$; AU = 0.61, $p < 0.01$). A strong association was observed between AU and SA (0.55, $p < 0.01$) and PRO was strongly associated with PL (0.50, $p < 0.05$).

TABLE 3.2 Frequencies Analysis Sample ($N = 22$)

Variable	Percentage
Age*	66.0 (13.4)
Male	9.1
Female	90.9
Veteran	31.8
Affiliated	36.4
General Member	31.8

Note: *Mean and SD for age.

TABLE 3.3 Correlations between Pre–Test Constructs

	AU	EM	PG	PRO	PL	SA
AU	1	0.44*	0.61**	0.23	0.08	0.55**
EM	0.44*	1	0.72**	0.64**	0.65**	0.78**
PG	0.61**	0.72**	1	0.57**	0.64**	0.59**
PRO	0.23	0.64**	0.57**	1	0.50*	0.53**
PL	0.08	0.65**	0.64**	0.50*	1	0.41
SA	0.55**	0.78**	0.59**	0.53	0.41	1

Note: $*p < 0.05$; $**p < 0.01$.
AU = Autonomy; **EM** = Environmental Mastery; **PG** = Personal Growth; **PRO** = Personal Relation with Others; **PL** = Purpose in Life; and **SA** = Self-acceptance.

TABLE 3.4 Internal Consistency

Construct	α
Autonomy	0.72
Environmental Mastery	0.84
Personal Growth	0.76
Relations with Others	0.78
Purpose in Life	0.70
Self-Acceptance	0.87

Correlations between constructs were strong as were tests of internal consistency, suggesting that the scales are reliable measures (Table 3.4). Although some items within a scale were observed to have a low corrected item score, no scale's alpha was significantly improved by removing test items, further validating the reliability of each construct scale. For instance, two items within AU (#2 and #20) were observed to have low corrected item scores (0.24 and 0.21); however, removing these items from the scale would minimally increase alpha from 0.72 to 0.73. As displayed in Table 3.4, each scale has an alpha greater than 0.70. Two scales, EM and SA, have alpha greater than 0.80.

Results

A paired sample t-test was conducted to compare the psychological well-being before and after participation in a Legacy Group experience. Overall, the psychological well-being scores improved for persons who participated in the group intervention. This improvement was due to the observed increase in mean difference scores for two constructs (Table 3.5). Average PG increased by nearly 2 points as there was a significant difference (X difference = 1.91, SD = 4.10) in the post–test and pre–test scores $t(21) = 2.18$, $p < 0.04$, and average PL scores

TABLE 3.5 Paired Sample *t*-Test: Constructs of PWB

Construct	X (SD)	Confidence intervals (CI) of difference	t
AU	1.18 (3.54)	0.39, 2.75	1.57
EM	0.02 (4.22)	−1.89, 1.85	−0.03
PG	1.91 (4.10)	3.73, 0.09	2.18*
PRO	0 (4.80)	−2.13, 2.13	0
PL	2.18 (3.79)	3.86, 0.50	2.70**
SA	−0.16 (4.26)	−2.05, 1.73	−0.18

Note: df = 21; *$p < 0.05$; **$p < 0.01$.
AU = Autonomy; **EM** = Environmental Mastery; **PG** = Personal Growth; **PRO** = Personal Relation with Others; **PL** = Purpose in Life; and **SA** = Self-acceptance.

increased by more than 2 points as there was a significant difference (X difference = 2.18, SD = 3.79) in post and pre-test scores $t(21) = 2.70$, $p < 0.01$. Results suggest that participation in the Legacy Groups significantly enhances PG and PL for members. Legacy Group facilitators reported that group members shared that they experienced improvement in their life direction and sense of meaning (PL). Overall, participants reported an increase in their openness to change and willingness to confront new challenges; they reported improvement in the ongoing development of their true self. Legacy Group members had a positive impact on members' self-confidence and how they believed they were viewed by others. Finally, independent *t*-tests were constructed to assess relationships between age, gender, member status, and individual test items of well-being. Results suggest that the general participants are more likely to have confidence in even their uncommon opinions after participating in a Legacy Group, compared to those similar veteran and affiliated members.

Lessons Learned

The purpose of the research study was to assess the efficacy of the Legacy Model. Overall, the Legacy Group intervention improved the psychological well-being of the study participants, specifically in the areas of PG and PL. Although measurement and study limitations exist, the results suggest that the Legacy Group intervention is both effective and relevant in improving the psychological well-being of group members.

References

American Group Psychotherapy Association. (2015). *Evidenced-based practice in group psychotherapy*. www.agpa.org/home/practice-resources/evidence-based-practice-in-group-psychotherapy

American Psychological Association. (2019). *Growing mental and behavioral health concerns facing older Americans.* www.apa.org/advocacy/health/older-americans-mental-behavioral-health

The American Psychological Association Guidelines. (2021). *Professional practice guidelines for evidence-based psychological practice in health care.* www.apa.org/about/policy/evidence-based-psychological-practice-health-care.pdf

American Psychological Association, Presidential Task Force on Evidence-Based Practice. (2006). Evidence-based practice in psychology. *American Psychologist, 61*(4), 271–285. https://doi.org/10.1037/0003-066X.61.4.271

Bergeron, C. D., & Smith, M. L. (2018). The impact of physical challenges on mental health of the aging population. In D. Maller & K. Langsam (Eds.), *The Praeger handbook of mental health; mental health and the aging community* (pp. 63–85). Praeger.

Ryff, C. D. (1989). Happiness is everything, or is it? Explorations on the meaning of psychological well-being. *Journal of Personality and Social Psychology, 57*(6), 1069–1081.

Ryff, C. D. (2014). Psychological well-being revisited: Advances in the science and practice of eudaimonia. *Psychotherapy and Psychosomatics, 83,* 10–28. https://doi.org/10.1159/000353263

Seifert, T. (2005). *The Ryff scales of psychological well-being.* Center of Inquiry at Wabash College. https://centerofinquiry.org/uncategorized/ryff-scales-of-psychological-well-being/

United States Department of Health & Human Services. (2022). *Healthy people 2030.* www.health.gov/healthypeople

Vaillant, G. E. (1993). *The wisdom of the ego.* Harvard University Press.

4

SERENDIPITY IN LEGACY WORK

When we began our work conducting Legacy Groups, we found specific claims of uncanny coincidences by individuals researching their ancestors and family history intriguing. We learned early on that it is not unusual for individuals seeking to learn about their ancestral legacy to report strange coincidences that often lead to a hint or new information in their legacy exploration. It has been described as a "bigger than us," "been here before," and "what are the chances," thoughts, and feelings. These occurrences can be powerful and surprisingly eerie. Fortunately, they are also, by definition, welcomed and happy experiences referred to as serendipity.

Within this chapter, we aim to prepare Legacy Group facilitators in understanding and assisting group members who share serendipitous experiences. Definitions of serendipity are provided and descriptions of the etymological history to explain the several types of serendipity that are purported to exist are reviewed. To assist readers in understanding serendipity and its relevance in legacy work, one of many conceptual models is offered. Most helpful in comprehending serendipity is to read the stories through the memory of the authors. All names used are fictitious.

Defining Serendipity

Jones (1993) published *Psychic Roots: Serendipity and Intuition in Genealogy* to share with the world experiences of "serendipity; events that happen simultaneously with no apparent causal connection but with deep significance for those who experience them" (p xii). Theresa had a series of strange coincidences after visiting a psychic. The psychic identified her passion for writing and told her that someone very close to her is supportive of her interest in writing. Intrigued at

DOI: 10.4324/9781003298168-5

the time, then the thought passed. Two days later, however, Theresa found an old picture of her grandmother in her daughter's room. She loved the old black and white photo for its simplicity, as it was one of her favorites. Her Gram passed away five years ago and they had been very close. Although she could not explain how the picture got there, she let her daughter keep the photograph near her bedside. The following day she experienced an uncomfortable boredom that was becoming all too familiar. She rifled through her bookcase seeking inspiration or at least distraction when suddenly an old letter fell to the floor. Tears came to her eyes as Theresa read her Gram's words written many years ago. She continued to miss her Gram deeply. She took pictures of both the photograph and the letter and shared them on Facebook with a post describing her experiences to share with the world. Theresa's story continued to unfold. She noticed a memorial card from her grandmother's funeral placed conspicuously on the television stand and again shared her experience on Facebook.

A series of coincidences or strange feelings are common experiences of serendipity. Throughout literature phrases such as "a happy accident," the "finding of things without seeking them," "any pleasant surprise," and a "discovery of something not sought" are used (de Rond, 2014). Similar words from definitions can be found in both *Merriam-Webster* and the *English Oxford Living* dictionaries.

Etymological History

The *Travels and Adventures of Three Princes of Serendip* was published by Michael Tramezzino in 1557. The tale contains many adventures involving three princes who had been sent out into the kingdom to expand their already vast knowledge. The most well-known tale involves a lost camel. In this tale, the princes are approached by a man on the road who enquires about his missing camel. The princes had not actually seen the man's camel but were able to describe it in detail: blind in one eye, missing a tooth, and lame. They offer even further specifics: the camel is carrying butter on one side and honey on the other, and it is being ridden by a pregnant woman. Because of their statements, the camel owner accuses them of stealing his camel and the princes are taken to the emperor to be charged. When questioned, the princes declare their innocence and explain that their knowledge about the camel was obvious:

- Grass was eaten on only one side of the road = the camel was blind in one eye
- Large cuds of chewed grass were on the road = a space as large as a missing tooth
- Only three hoof tracks were visible with the trace of a dragged foot = lame
- Trail of ants, flies = seek fat, honey
- Small footprints, strong smell of urine, hands used to help up = pregnant rider

The princes are not punished but instead remain with the emperor and continue to impress him with their observational skills. Although the story was written in 1557, it was not until 200 years later, on January 28, 1754, that Horace Walpole referenced it in a letter to his friend and cousin, Horace Mann, to describe a personal experience for which he could find no words. Walpole used the word "serendipity" to compare his recent experience to that of the Princes of Serendip. Like him, he wrote, the princes had traveled about "making discoveries, by accidents and sagacity, of things which they were not in quest of" (Merton & Barber, 2004, p. 2). Ironically, he is considered the creator of the term and the first to use it. Although he defined serendipity as the accidental sagacity of information not originally sought, the princes do not ever discover anything. Instead, they make repeated deductions based on keen observations. The princes have an ability to identify and match pieces of seemingly unrelated information in a meaningful way and apply it with purpose.

Either of these definitions (i.e., happy accident; chance coupled with sagacity) would be sufficient for those of us experiencing them in their subtle, sometimes creepy, yet beneficial ways. But empirical research rarely settles for sufficient, and so it may come as no surprise that researchers have created operational definitions and conceptual models to better understand serendipity. They have measured, analyzed, and presented all sorts of serendipity data. Unfortunately, instead of simplifying the concept, it appears that their attempts have only muddied the serendipity waters.

Types of Serendipity

Serendipity stories vary in degree of strange, happy, and often opportunistic. Austin (2003) believed that there were four serendipity types, distinguishable by how much involvement the individual had on the event. The first two, Blind Luck and Happy Accident, require different degrees of chance. Two additional types require chance, as well as an active cognitive component: Prepared Mind and Individual Characteristics.

Blind Luck Serendipity involves just that, with no real intention from the individual, but a feeling of being at the right place at the right time. For example, Lou's search for information regarding his birth mother's family history led him, accompanied by his wife, to his maternal grandparent's burial place. Lou knew little about this part of his family and was excited at the prospect of learning about his birth mother. Strangely, when Lou traveled to an unfamiliar state and crossed the town line, he found himself in front of the cemetery he was seeking. Stranger still, as Lou went on, he said that he observed a mother and daughter planting flowers at a grave, seemingly oblivious to the gentle rain. The mother looked up and asked if Lou needed assistance, whereby he replied that he was looking for a particular family plot. The woman was clearly touched and informed Lou that she was a member of that family. He found a cousin in the cemetery that day! A serendipitous moment indeed.

Gertrude shared a similar Blind Luck, supposed to be experience. It all began when she learned there was someone interested in one of her historical paintings displayed at a recent art museum show. The specific piece was of an old theater she had visited while traveling, but she learned that the buyer could not afford the piece as priced. The prospective buyer was the art museum accountant. Apparently, the accountant had received tickets to the art show and invited her aunt and uncle. The now older couple had once been this theater's operators for 40 years! You can imagine their surprise when they saw the painting. The painting had great emotional value to them, and their niece wanted to purchase it for their upcoming 50th wedding anniversary. Gertrude shared that after hearing how the couple came to see the painting, she felt compelled to adjust the price. She was happy to report that the painting now resides in what she believes is its true home.

According to Austin's (2003) framework, it was Blind Luck that landed Lou at the correct cemetery on the same day that a relative was also there, just as it was Blind Luck that brought an aged couple to a museum show displaying art of the very theater they operated for over 40 years. But whereas Blind Luck Serendipity is due to chance events that occur with no effort from the observer, Happy Accidents occur when an observer directly impacts those chance events as this next story explains.

Sharon and her father were at a cemetery placing flags and bronzed placards for deceased members of her family who were military veterans. Her father took a break to accept a phone call, while Sharon went to work conducting the task at hand. She noticed many other flags and adornments needing adjusting, so she busied herself from plot to plot straightening crooked placards and leaning flags. After several plots, she was amazed to note the name on a particular gravestone was familiar. As her father was conveniently speaking on the phone to her aunt, who also had interest in family genealogy, Sharon inquired about the individual's name on the stone. She learned from her aunt that she was related to that individual. She was excited about discovering a new family line right there in the graveyard that day.

Austin (2003) purports that Happy Accident Serendipity involves chance, and Sharon's story contains plenty of it: stumbling upon family gravestones and having her genealogy-savvy aunt accessible on the phone. But her experience was also a direct result of her behavioral choices: to fix the flags and adornments in the cemetery. Austin's framework also references two types of serendipity that require a cognitive component, and Lou and Sharon stories depict Prepared Mind and Individual Characteristics Serendipity. Lou had engaged in independent research before making the journey to the cemetery. Having only a birth name to start with, he considered it a small miracle finding his mother's death record on the internet. Armed with this tidbit, however, he learned of her age and cause of death, and the names of his birth parents and potential burial spots. Lou hoped that his mother would also be buried there. It was hope and blind luck that landed Lou at the right cemetery on that day, but only a Prepared Mind could have set him on the path he took.

A good example of an individual characteristic that revolves around a specific area or interest that Austin (2003) contends are serendipity-prone is Sharon's experience. Her individual characteristic led to raised awareness to the crooked flags and moved her to walk around adjusting them and the other military adornments. Further, she had a joint interest in genealogical research that she had shared with her aunt for many years. Although she may had come across new gravestones on that particular day, her own distinct, individual characteristics played an important role in both her increased awareness and her ability to apply the information presented to her.

Liestman (1992) offered a more expansive framework as he gave separate credence to the seemingly chance events performed by the unseen or unknown, and this aspect resonates in many of the stories shared with us. Yolander had recently lost her mother when she found an old autograph book that belonged to her mother and began looking through it. In it she found a message to her mother from her mother's grandmother. It was written during the Christmas holiday long ago when her mother was worried about her own brother who was serving overseas in World War II. This type of opportunistic discovery is what Liestman (1992) referred to as serendipity by Prevenient Grace. One has to query her great-grandmother's intention to speak to her and offer her strength and hope during a difficult time.

Serendipity by Prevenient Grace can occur without warning, as Yolander experienced. Other times those events are exactly what you asked, or even prayed, for as with Anna. She was getting close to uncovering a long-held family secret. She shared that although some family members had theories about this secret, no one presented facts. Sharon, Anna's sister, believed that an aged maternal grandmother had important clues to offer. Unfortunately, whenever asked, the grandmother would conveniently forget, avoid, or not hear the question. But recently, Anna felt that with the advancement in DNA testing she was certain she could obtain the answers she desperately wanted. She sought out her stored family history material, and yet no information was to be found! Everything she had acquired from pictures and documents and genograms was missing. She was certain that everything was kept in a black zippered binder and tore her office and home apart in the hunt for her material. Exhausted and frustrated, she made a promise to the heavens to no longer dig into the family secret if only she could locate her legacy material. She found her binder in what she considered a very illogical place and was puzzled when it was red not black in color as she had remembered! Anna has since kept her promise and left the family secret just that. Anna knew what the binder looked like and where to look for it, but it was not until she made her heavenly pact that she was able to locate the material. According to Liestman (1992), unseen forces directed her to a different place containing the different-colored binder. Bittersweet, perhaps, and consistent with Liestman, the event was one of Serendipity by Prevenient Grace.

Van Andel (1994) offered yet another perspective. He embraced the definition the discovery of something not originally sought, yet believed serendipity came in positive, negative, and even pseudo types. Positive serendipity consists of an initial chance event followed by further investigation (i.e., sagacity), whereas negative serendipity consists of the chance event with no follow-up study (no cognitive component). Pseudoserendipity occurs when chance events lead to the discovery of something that had been originally sought.

Heidi's honeymoon cruise experience is quite compelling. While relaxing at the pool, she noticed that another couple lying in the sun had fallen asleep. She was concerned about them getting sunburned, but also worried about the appropriateness of covering strangers with towels. She decided to cover them and woke them in the process. This led to a conversation with the couple and Heidi learned that they had been married on the same day and were headed to the same island. They agreed to meet and were able to enjoy many activities together. Upon leaving, they all made the promise to stay in touch. The couples recently celebrated their 30 years of friendship. They initially met by chance and then became two of Heidi's best friends. This was an unsought chance meeting. The couple's commitment to stay connected over the years (i.e., sagacity) created what Van Andel (1994) deems positive serendipity.

Midge's experience offers an example of negative serendipity, not to suggest her story ends badly! Van Andel (1994) suggests negative serendipity is also a happy chance event that was not sought, but one that occurs from little effort from the observer. Midge quite literally walked into it or onto it. Her experience is about a random walk one day. During the walk, she glanced down and noticed that children had been making chalk drawings on the blacktop. She continued to walk and looked at the art until one piece caused her to stop. Someone had written a brief quote about legacy. Midge had just finished communicating with a colleague about this very topic. She took a picture of the text believing that she may want to use it in the future. The brief quote: "Legacy, what is a legacy? It's the planting of seeds in a garden you get to see."

Pseudoserendipity is when the observer has been seeking information but comes to find it via chance events. We can return to Sharon who was straightening flags in the cemetery and came across a new family line. She clearly found something she was often seeking in her genealogical information. Although on this day, she was not actively conducting research. Instead, she accidently found new family gravestones while engaged in a different task. Consider though, her lifework prepared her to embrace the significance of the event.

Explaining Serendipity

Serendipity is often used synonymously with gut feeling or intuition. Barbara had a gut feeling experience in late February 1970 when she was a junior in nursing school. Barbara's parents did not visit during the week and her boyfriend was in the marines serving in Vietnam, yet this night she repeatedly got up from her desk and went to her window as if expecting someone or something. She had an uncomfortable, agitated feeling she could not name or extinguish. Sometime later the next day she heard her best friend paged for a phone call. When her friend entered Barbara's room she was crying, yet Barbara felt strangely peaceful. Barbara was told that her boyfriend had been wounded, was being sent home, and her parents were on their way to her now. Her sense of calm was initially perceived as shock by many, but Barbara believed her response was a result of her knowing her boyfriend's journey home had commenced.

Déjà vu

Serendipity as a strange feeling is sometimes compared to *déjà vu*, but the two are indeed different. *Déjà vu* is French for already seen and is responsible for that strange "I have been here before," "haven't we met," sensation. All men and women, of all ages, experience *déjà vu*, but it is mostly reported by those aged 15–25 years (Bartolomei et al., 2012). Science suggests that *déjà vu* may result from changes in dopamine levels, commonly experienced in this age group. Individuals with medial temporal lobe epilepsy often report intense *déjà vu* before a seizure, experiences referred to as auras. This type of seizure activity involves the hippocampus, which regulates both short- and long-term memories. Research suggests that neuronal misfiring in the hippocampus of these individuals and healthy individuals can impact the formation of memory and help explain the sensation of familiarity that occurs with *déjà vu* (Jones, 1993; Martin et al., 2012; Taiminen & Jääskeläinen, 2001). Although serendipity and *déjà vu* have similar aspects, these are clearly different experiences. *Déjà vu* is likely the result of neuronal misfiring, therefore, the result of neurobiological processes within an individual. Serendipity is the result of an interaction between an observer and the observed.

Serendipity Research Models

One method researchers use to help others understand a complex idea is to create a conceptual model. Agarwal (2015) suggested that serendipity was an important and missing part of the past models. As such, he created a model that allowed space for serendipity as part of the larger process. According to his model, Information Searching involves a very specific interaction between an individual and a system to gain knowledge (i.e., library, internet). More broadly, Information

Seeking is based on the conscious effort to acquire information. Agarwal includes Serendipitous Information Finding (SIF) as a distinct concept that can occur during Seeking or Searching.

Consider the story of Veronica in which she made the conscious decision to engage in cemetery explorations with the hope of learning about her family ancestry. Her self-described sense of urgency, as if possessed, with this new quest certainly falls under Information Seeking. Her experience crosses into Information Searching as she drives around the cemetery, growing ever more frantic, searching for the family plot. A thought popped into her head to stop and make a call to the cemetery keeper for information. The phone number she had was to the person's home. Interestingly, the person was home as she had forgotten something that she needed for work. Veronica explained to the cemetery keeper that she was currently in the cemetery but was unable to locate the plot she had been searching for. Interestingly, the cemetery records were stored under the cemetery keeper's bed who then proceeded to give Veronica information regarding names, causes of death, and even residences of her ancestors. The most profound coincidence is when Veronica stated that she would like to view the family plot, the cemetery keeper instructed her to drive to the flagpole, the exact spot where Veronica had parked her car to make the phone call. The family plot was right there. Veronica was shocked at the eerie series of events. The cemetery keeper informed her to expect many more uncanny experiences throughout her legacy journey. Veronica's account is a great example of Seeking and Searching behavior that results in a serendipitous experience. Agarwal (2015) claims that serendipity can occur when an individual is engaged in non-purposeful seeking, as well. His model allows space for SIF in Other Information Behavior, suggesting that an individual may not be Seeking or Searching information yet may encounter it anyway.

Many well-known discoveries in science have been the result of keen deductive skills occurring after a chance event – in other words, serendipity. Some of these events have made our lives easier as with Velcro and Teflon. Other events could be argued to have made our lives more enjoyable as with Coca-Cola and cheese. Still other events have done nothing short of altering the history of the world as with Fleming (e.g., penicillin) and Richet (e.g., allergens). An understanding and openness to serendipity as a legitimate part of legacy work is critical to those on the journey. Similarly, your willingness to support and explore members' happy accidents makes for an easier and more enjoyable legacy process, a journey that for some may be nothing short of altering the history of their world.

References

Agarwal, N. K. (2015). Towards a definition of serendipity in information behavior. *Information Research, 20*(3), paper 675; *Journal of the History of the Neurosciences, 19*, 253–270.

Austin, J. H. (2003). *Chase, chance, and creativity: The lucky art of novelty.* The MIT Press.

Bartolomei, F., Barbeau E. J., Nguyen, T., McGonigal, A., Régis, J., Chauvel, P., & Wendling, F. (2012). Rhinal-hippocampal interactions during *déjà vu*. *Clinical Neurophysiology: Official Journal of the International Federation of Clinical Neurophysiology, 123*(3), 489–495.

de Rond, M. (2014). The structure of serendipity. *Culture and Organization, 20*(5), 342–358.

Jones, H. (1993). *Psychic roots: Serendipity and intuition in genealogy*. Genealogical Publishing Co., Inc.

Liestman, D. (1992). Chance in the midst of design: Approaches to library research serendipity. *RQ, 31*(4), 524–532. www.jstor.org/stable/25829128

Martin, C., Mirsattari, S., Pruessner, J., Pietrantonio, S., Burneo, J., Hayman-Abello, B., & Köhler, S. (2012, November). *Déjà vu* in unilateral temporal-lobe epilepsy is associated with selective familiarity impairments on experimental tasks of recognition memory. *Neuropsychologia, 50*(13), 2981–2991.

Merton, R., & Barber, E. (2004). *The travels and adventures of serendipity*. Princeton University Press.

Taiminen, T., & Jääskeläinen, S. K. (2001, September). Intense and recurrent *déjà vu* experiences related to amantadine and phenylpropanolamine in a healthy male. *Journal of Clinical Neuroscience, 8*(5), 460–462.

Van Andel, P. (1994, June). Anatomy of the unsought finding. Serendipity: Origin, history, domains, traditions, appearances, patterns and programmability. *The British Journal for the Philosophy of Science, 45*(2), 631–648.

PART II

Legacy Group Curriculum in Action

Part II: The Legacy Group Curriculum in Action provides an in-depth look at the two different formats of the Legacy Group curriculum. The original curriculum was designed as a process group. That is, facilitators used therapeutic group exercises to encourage self-reflection, to enhance self-awareness of members, and to foster cohesion in a safe environment. The goal was to assist the members in identifying how group members wished to explore and/or preserve their legacy and facilitate the process of meaning-making. Over time, groups were offered to a wider and more diverse population. The modifications offered to community-dwelling adults would clearly not suffice for older adults with physical disabilities and cognitive impairments. In response to these needs, a second curriculum, Activity-Based Legacy Group Curriculum, was developed for adults residing in assisted-living or skilled care settings who would benefit from added structure, guidance, and support.

Both the Process-Focused Legacy Group Curriculum (Chapter 5) and the Activity-Based Legacy Group Curriculum (Chapter 6) are presented in detail. Due to the nature of the population served, differences in delivery will be noted from screening processes through each of the three phases of the group experience. The core of the Legacy Model remains constant for both delivery formats. Chapter 7, Clinical Reflections, is a personal and reflective collection of facilitator memories with three different populations: *Women Who Served*, *Adults in Search of Meaning*, and *Older Adults on a Journey*. The book closes with Chapter 8, Potential Audiences, Challenges, and Special Considerations, for practitioners interested in conducting Legacy Groups and Legacy Workshops with other populations as well as some best practice guidance.

DOI: 10.4324/9781003298168-6

PART II
Legacy Group Curriculum in Action

5

PROCESS-FOCUSED LEGACY GROUP CURRICULUM

The original intention of the Legacy Model was to conduct process groups using therapeutic activities are provided that have been shown to be highly effective with facilitating self-reflection, building a sense of community and legacy exploration and preservation with group members. Over time it became apparent that a process group curriculum worked well with high functioning adults. As such, the authors created a second group curriculum which is reviewed in the next chapter. The Process-Focused Legacy Group Curriculum is broken down into detailed steps. With each step, examples are provided from the memory of Legacy Group facilitators. Examples use pseudo names.

Pre-Group Screening

The screening protocol involves a pre-group meeting with prospective members. Facilitators provide an overview of Legacy Groups and explain how groups function. Prospective members are given an opportunity to share their personal understanding of legacy and what they expect to get from and offer to the group. Their readiness (i.e., cognitive, physical, emotional) and interest in legacy exploration are assessed during this initial rapport-building meeting. In addition, their understanding of the ways in which they can become keepers of the meaning are explored. Potential group members are screened directly and indirectly for factors that may affect their ability to participate in a Process-Focused Legacy Group experience. Individuals observed to have physical and/or cognitive limitations are not deterred from joining a group; instead, facilitators have the option to adjust and make modifications to the curriculum or recommend to prospective members to join an Activity-Based Legacy Group. Screening meetings are also used to provide prospective members with all required documents and consent forms.

DOI: 10.4324/9781003298168-7

Phase I: A Supportive Group Environment and Realistic Goal Setting

Phase I of Process-Focused Legacy Groups entails creating a safe and supportive group environment that will be fostered and maintained throughout the life of the group experience. The foundation that is built during these early weeks is critical for members to feel safe to explore and share openly. Brief icebreakers during these early sessions can be used to assist in getting to know one another more deeply. Therapeutic exercises that are brief and facilitate each member's ability, desire to reflect, and freely share is beneficial to the group process. Providing a writing prompt, then having the group members journal, and finally share their written work is an example of a process-focused therapeutic exercise used for exploring individual goals for legacy work as well as for enhancing cohesion. One true and tried therapeutic exercise is asking members to quickly write ten legacy words, ideas, or themes on a sheet of paper. Next, members are instructed to close their eyes briefly. Upon opening them, they are asked to scan their list and circle the item that grabs their attention and write about this concept or idea for three to five minutes. Last, group members volunteer to read what they wrote or share an overview. This exercise provides a vehicle for sharing legacy experiences that helps build a supportive and safe group environment.

Building a strong supportive group environment is important for members to feel comfortable before creating legacy goals. A word of caution: goals set too high are difficult to meet and goals set too low have been shown to lower motivation and investment. Further, all members benefit from writing down their goals, including one or two benchmarks, if applicable. Asking members to share their goals will serve in both solidifying the members' understanding of what they will be undertaking and strengthening connections between group members. Be advised that unless a facilitator teaches realistic goal setting, it is not uncommon for members to arrive with bags of photos from their attic and a quest to organize them all in one day. Each session closes with the opportunity for members to reflect on the session as well as how their experience will be assimilated into their understanding and perspective of their legacy.

Week 1

Introductions: Allow ample time for members to introduce themselves to the other group members. This is an opportunity to share experiences of past or current interest with legacy exploration. What brought them here? What do they expect from this group experience?

Provide Legacy Group overview: It is important to provide group members with an overview of the group experience, including delivery format, meeting times, and expectations so that the members have a clear understanding of the purpose and format of the group. This is a good time to collect contact information and have a protocol in place for late or missed group sessions.

Review Legacy Group expectations: A conversation about confidentiality and respect for all members is essential to a successful group experience. Suggest that members often get out of the group equal to the effort and investment they put in; therefore, full participation is recommended.

Legacy-themed icebreaker: Some members respond well to exercises that help jump-start the getting-to-know-you phase. One example of a guided exercise is to have members share a favorite childhood memory.

Process legacy ideas and identify potential goals: Some members may come to group with several, large and completely unrealistic ideas. Others will come with nothing and stare blankly. Both are common at this stage and are part of the initial group process. Suggest that members with a plethora of ideas share one or two; their excitement and creativity are often highly contagious! Validate group members who do not have an idea or goal in mind. Check in with them after the others have shared to see if any shared legacy exploration or preservation ideas and/or goals sparked an idea for them. See Appendix II for legacy project ideas to share with the group members.

Complete necessary forms: Complete the informed consent and other forms during this session.

Closing reflections: Members are given an opportunity to reflect and share thoughts and feelings related to this group session. Will this group experience provide an opportunity to explore their legacy and foster meaning-making?

Jana joined a Legacy Group at her local senior center. She recently retired from an administrative position at a large insurance company. As she introduced herself, she shared that she was adjusting to the changes in her life due to experiencing less pressure as she no longer had a hectic schedule that involved commuting and a long day of work negotiating many responsibilities. Exploring her legacy sounded appealing to her as she often thought about researching her ancestry and organizing family photos. She presented as a well-organized and goal-oriented person. Jana was soft-spoken, articulate, and attentively listened to other group members as they shared their stories during the first session. She expressed surprise when she learned that members would not be researching genealogy. Her interest seemed to peak when thinking about a project related to her family photos.

Week 2

Check-in: What have members been reflecting about over the past week? What did their first Legacy Group experience offer them or bring up for them? Any changes or shifts in perspective?

Legacy prompt: Journaling with a prompt allows members an opportunity to write, share, and give feedback to others. *Creating a Spiritual Legacy* by Daniel

Taylor offers therapeutic exercises, prompts, and questions for self-reflection. One example from Taylor's book is, "[W]hat can I pass on to others that will make their lives better or easier or deeper?" (2011). This is an excellent way to invite members to share and enhance the group process.

Goal setting: Some group members may be familiar with writing goals, but others may not. Explain that we often create goals in our mind; yet these goals remain abstract and, therefore, more difficult to attain. Writing out clearly defined goals can be challenging and even more frustrating than one might expect. Facilitators can offer guidance and support by asking clarifying questions and helping each member by assisting them in identifying realistic expectations. Introduce the concept of creating benchmarks that serve as a staircase to reaching a goal. It is helpful if each step is clearly defined and realistic. A discussion involving SMART goals is beneficial. Create goals that are: Specific, Measurable, Attainable, Realistic, and Time-bound.

Example: *Before goal-setting experience*: I want to organize all my family photographs.

Example: *After goal-setting experience*: I will organize three packages of photographs by theme per week for 10 weeks.

Benchmark One: For our next group meeting, I will have a space dedicated to my legacy project and have made a list of supplies (e.g., tape, scissors, pens).

Benchmark Two: Within two weeks, I will have six packages of photos labeled and I will have identified categories (e.g., summer, grandkids, friends, travel, holiday).

Closing reflections: Members are given an opportunity to reflect and share. How do they see the group experience impacting their personal journey? How will goal setting assist their process of meaning-making? What are the next steps? What might help?

Jana shared in group that she joined a Legacy Group with plans to complete a large genealogy project. After some reflection and reviewing her notes, she began thinking about projects that involved family photos. Having the opportunity to share her ideas in group, then to self-reflect, she realized that she was pushing herself as if she was still working at her job! She shared in the group that she felt a sense of relief realizing that she was on her own timeclock. This was the beginning of a new chapter in her life. This group was an opportunity for her to engage in self-directed activities on her own timeline. With reflection and feedback from group members, she decided to slowly discover what was in one box of photos. In the end, she decided to approach her legacy exploration with curiosity and temperance.

Week 3

Check-in: What have the members' experiences been like over the past week? How have they made sense of the previous group session? Any thoughts about their goals? How are members feeling about sharing project ideas and their progress in group?

Legacy exercise: The facilitator may sense that the group process moves effortlessly without an exercise to prompt members. Other groups may benefit from an exercise to facilitate the process and provide guidance with member sharing.

Share project ideas: Members are encouraged to share their project ideas in the format of a realistic goal with one or two benchmarks. Stress that the group is here to provide guidance and support. Reassure members that progress is not measured in quantity. It is about the significance and personal meaning associated with their legacy journey.

Closing reflections: What was it like to share your legacy exploration or project? What was it like to listen to feedback about your legacy from group members? Have you encountered challenges along your journey?

By the third week of the group, Jana was visibly more relaxed. During the check-in, she shared that she selected one random box and had begun to look at the photos. She took the advice offered from the group last week to simply review all the photos before engaging in the process of identifying family members and organizing them. Jana shared that she was astonished to learn that hours had passed while she was looking at family photos! A group member asked what the photos were of. Jana shared that they were photos of family vacations. She provided no further explanation. As usual, Jana continued to prompt others with her thoughtful questions about their own plans for a legacy project.

Phase II: Personal Legacy Work, Guidance, and Support

Phase II is the longest of the three phases and consists of seven sessions. Throughout these sessions, the facilitator balances the important task of continuing to build *cohesion* and *trust* within the group, while attending to each individual and the group as a whole. An important facilitator role is to help members stay in the *here-and-now* and validate each member's experience. Creating a safe and supportive environment inclusive of diversity often serves to encourage members to share during check-in and with closing reflections. The legacy work that occurs during the session consists of sharing experiences that arise while engaging in and working on individual legacy exploration and/or projects. Appendix II, Legacy Group Resources, provides a wealth of information and guidance for facilitators who would like to conduct a Legacy Group.

Weeks 4–10

Check-in: Although members may be excited or anxious to share or ask for guidance about their legacy exploration and/or project, it is important to allow time for check-in and maintain this sacred time for reflecting on their group experiences. There will be time in the group session to discuss their legacy work and seek guidance from other members.

Project updates: This is the time for members to share their progress on individual legacy work. Facilitators assist members with reflecting more deeply. Other members may use this time to discuss challenges encountered, surprises found, or accomplishments made.

Meaning-making process: This is where facilitators and group members engage in processing their experience and foster meaning-making with their legacy exploration and preservation experience. What does this mean to you? Are you feeling impacted or changed? How has your understanding of family, ancestry, or legacy changed or been validated?

Reflect on goals: Goals created earlier are often forgotten along the journey. When a group member feels distressed regarding lack of progress or branches off into multiple directions, the facilitator can ask the group for assistance in refocusing and reevaluating this member's initial goals. Providing an opportunity to reassess goals, legacy work status, and receive feedback is invaluable.

Closing reflections: What has most impacted you today? How do you see your exploration or project now? Has it changed since we began? Will you share your legacy work with others? How do you anticipate that it will be received? How does this legacy journey offer the opportunity to look backward and forward simultaneously?

Jana at times took on the role as guide and at other times engaged like a student in group. Her fellow group members grew to appreciate her ability to listen respectfully and formulate sensitive questions and comments. She oftentimes pointed out a strength or a success. She appeared to appreciate the support that she received from members as she shared about her journey when looking at photos from her past. A very touching experience occurred when the group facilitator led members in an activity using the Japanese poetry Haiku. Jana remembered learning about Haiku in her English class, yet had never written a poem using this technique. She easily constructed a poem and helped others construct theirs. In a later session she shared that she had lost her son in a motorcycle accident in California a few years earlier. Jana shared that she and her husband grieved in different ways. One wanted to process the loss; the other found conversation about their son too painful. While looking through boxes, she found a photo of her son. She left the photo on the kitchen counter with a Haiku poem that she wrote about him. A few days later, she found that her husband had written another Haiku. A lovely way to explore their grief and respect each other's process.

Phase III: Share, Review Goals, Next Steps, and Say Goodbye

During Phase III, group members share their legacy exploration and/or preservation projects and discuss any next steps that they are prepared to take in their journey. They celebrate their work and the legacy work of others. It is important to continue to maintain a safe and supportive environment that group members have come to know. Be mindful that due to the nature of the legacy exploration and/or projects, celebrating them may be difficult. Saying goodbye to the Legacy Group experience can be facilitated using group reflections about their overall experience. Many members acknowledge that their initial goals and first impressions appear worlds away. Although each individual session has offered opportunities to share regarding the ongoing process, the facilitator may shed light on the concept that the sum of the parts is not always equal to the whole. Now that the group experience is behind them, members will have the opportunity to view their experience from a very different perspective. Allow time for members to thank one another for their support and guidance, share before and after impressions and talk about their growth and report any changes in understanding of their place in their family, community, generation, and globally.

Week 11

Check-in: Continue opening each session by offering the opportunity to reflect on the previous group session.

Sharing of legacy exploration and/or projects and review goals: Members are given the opportunity to share their work with others. It is helpful to prompt members to share their experiences of their legacy exploration and/or project as well as the description of their work. Create a space for celebration and pride for those who are feeling ready and support for those who may need more time to assimilate this experience. Help members connect their legacy work with their goals and validate adjustments and changes that were made along the way.

Closing reflections: Prepare for closing the group experience. How are members feeling in the here-and-now? Feeling about themselves? What is it like to be ending the Legacy Group experience?

Week 12

Check-in: Routine and consistency are important as these help members to know what to expect and serve to support a safe environment that is critical to a successful group experience. What have members been thinking about over the past week, knowing that this is the last group session?

Consider next steps: Group members are given the opportunity to share their personal experience and to ask questions regarding potential next steps for themselves or about the legacy journey of other members. This discussion may spark ideas that may not have been previously considered. Allow ample time for this process.

Reflecting on the Legacy Group experience: This time is for members to reflect on the entire group experience. How are they different from how they were when the group began? What has contributed to this change? What did members notice about their interactions, relationships in or out of group? What did they notice about their journey while exploring or preserving their legacy? This is the last opportunity for meaning-making.

Closing group: Offer a last thank you and share your experience as the facilitator of this Legacy Group experience.

The Process-Focused Legacy Group curriculum was developed for high-functioning and motivated group members who express an interest in exploring and preserving some aspects of their legacy. Resources are provided to help prepare the facilitators interested in conducting Legacy Group. Appendix I Legacy Project Ideas and Appendix II Legacy Group Resources contain useful information.

Reference

Taylor, D. (2011). *Creating a spiritual legacy: How to share your stories, values, and wisdom* (p. 24). Brazos Press.

6

ACTIVITY-BASED LEGACY GROUP CURRICULUM

Chapter six provides an in-depth description of the Activity-Based Legacy Group curriculum. developed for older adults as well as individuals with physical disabilities and/or cognitive impairments. This curriculum can be easily adapted for children and adolescent Legacy Groups. Activities and legacy project ideas are provided to assist group facilitators with making accommodations while upholding the dignity of members when conducting groups with adults with diverse needs. Appendix II, Legacy Group Resources, contains information to assist facilitators in gaining knowledge about legacy exploration and preservation in group work.

Pre-Group Screening

Screening for an Activity-Based Legacy Group can be completed in a group meeting where the facilitator provides information about the Legacy Group experience. Individuals are encouraged to participate by asking questions, sharing stories, and offering their own perspectives regarding legacy and how they might be a keeper of the meaning. Icebreaker activities may include oral journaling or creating Haiku poetry together. These initial group member screenings allow sufficient assessment and identification of physical disabilities and/or cognitive impairments that may need accommodations and support during the Legacy Group experience.

Phase I: A Supportive Group Environment and Setting Realistic Goals

Phase I of the Activity-Based Legacy Group involves the creation of a safe and supportive group environment. Weeks 1–3 consist of therapeutic activities that

DOI: 10.4324/9781003298168-8

function as icebreakers, rapport builders, and process drivers. Like Process-Focused Legacy Groups, members will create realistic goals around exploring and preserving their legacy. Members in Activity-Based Legacy Groups often do not create or complete long-term projects, yet many of the activities conducted in this curriculum are easily adaptable for developing a longer-term project. For example, a group member may begin by writing a single letter to a grandchild during a group session. This experience may spark the idea of a long-term personal legacy project that entails writing regularly to their grandchild.

The Activities Director of an assisted-living facility, who had great insight into the abilities and needs of their residents, selected some residents for a pre-screening meeting. As a way of introducing Legacy Groups to members, the facilitator decided to have residents construct a collage that reminded them of a favorite experience in their life. Poster board, markers, scissors, glue, and different types of magazines were provided. Most of the residents engaged in the activity without hesitation. They began sharing pictures, headlines, and memories. Personal stories emerged that highlighted their individual legacies. Ms. S was flipping through magazines, not certain how to proceed. One of the residents began talking with her, offering her magazines while drawing attention to images of flowers. The kindness and support of one group member provided the bridge to a successful activity for Ms. S, as she had early onset dementia. As facilitators, we became aware that this woman would need support and encouragement to participate in a group experience. It was evident that residents had differing levels of cognitive capacity, physical ability, and confidence. This activity provided residents with the opportunity to share lived experiences and memorable stories from the past. What emerged was the beginning of a Legacy Group.

Week 1: Group Activities for Introductions and Rapport Building

Activity – Making Note of Your Legacy

Materials: Paper and pens.

Description: Members are informed that they will be given a brief prompt to which they will write for three minutes. It is important to recommend that they not overthink, instead, free write. Request that group members write continuously for the allotted time even if they believe they are finished.

Prompt: The word family conjures up many images, thoughts, and emotions for people. Certainly, this is because the word, as well as the experience of family, means different things to different people. Over the next three minutes, please describe your understanding of the word and experience of family.

Therapeutic intent: A variety of different prompts could be used. With this theme-based prompt, members are invited to process similarities and differences within the group. It is helpful for the facilitator to encourage members to consider how these are known and how they might be passed down through families, cultures, and through the generations.

Week 2: Legacy Activity to Delve More Deeply

Activity – Digging Up Words

Materials: Large poster board and colored markers.

Description: This activity is a group acrostic. The facilitator writes the word LEGACY from top to bottom on the left side of the poster board. Then, the facilitator asks the group to brainstorm words that begin with the letter L that relate to the word LEGACY. Each word a group member contributes is written next to the corresponding letter. The facilitator will continue with each letter until the acrostic is complete. This poster can be brought to each group meeting to remind members how they attributed meaning to the term LEGACY and may serve to spark further discussion.

Therapeutic Intent: This is a brainstorming activity that encourages creativity and thought expansion about what is associated with legacy. Some members may hear words offered that spark new associations for them that were not initially considered.

Options: Facilitators used a variety of different words in this exercise: legacy, family, history, ancestry, and so on.

LEGACY acrostic: The LEGACY activity began slowly. As more abstract thinking and connections began to flow, the activity moved more quickly than I could move my pen! There was much laughter as members tried to explain their rational for their words. C for Crustacean resulted in a moment of complete silence before the room broke out in laughter. This member explained that her husband had created a tradition in their family that began when their grandchildren were very young. The tradition involved inviting family members over for lobster night. The children always enjoyed racing their lobsters before eating them. We were exhausted from laughing and on the fourth pass of the acrostic, we went with Crustacean for C. This was a wonderful way to hear snippets of personal legacy experiences and have members bond together around shared memories and laughter.

Week 3: Increase Cohesion Activity

Activity – Question Ball Activity

Materials: Light, medium-sized inflatable ball and markers.

Description: The facilitator writes questions on the ball (i.e., imagine a soccer ball). Members toss the ball to one another or roll it across the table. Group members must read aloud the question where their right thumb lands when the ball is caught and then answer the question. Consider questions that may serve as appropriate icebreaker prompts: favorite childhood memory, describe your first job, or where were you born or grew up? Ever travel outside of the country? Did you have a pet as a child?

Therapeutic Intent: This activity is conducted early in the Activity-Based Legacy Group experience and serves to enhance rapport. The questions are nonthreatening and foster cohesion as group members share common experiences. As processing occurs, stimulation of memory often sparks new levels of conversation among members.

As with any therapeutic group, members will spend these first weeks grappling internally (and sometimes externally) with existential questions, such as "Why am I here?" "What am I supposed to accomplish?" "What is my purpose?" The role of the facilitator is to validate the members' queries, to lower anxiety associated with existential factors and to express that all diverse ways of thinking and believing are welcomed.

Phase II: Personal Legacy Work, Guidance, and Support

Phase II covers weeks 4–10 of the group experience. Members have become familiar with each other and have begun to build relationships. Members are exploring their legacy more deeply as they engage in various legacy activities. In addition, some members work on their own projects with the assistance of family members, aids, or the activity director. Legacy activities incorporate rapport building and reflective components to best support the members on this journey. Facilitators observe group process to ensure all members participate at their most comfortable and safe level. Phase II is the longest section of the group experience. Group activities are used to strengthen *cohesion*, while offering an opportunity to reflect on concepts of their personal legacy.

Activity – Personal Legacy Artifacts

Materials: Ask group members to bring in memorabilia or a nostalgic item to the group (e.g., piece of jewelry, a book, coins, a mug or vase, or photo).

Description: Ask the group members to share the story of the item and their future intentions for the piece.

Therapeutic Intent: This activity is a powerful and moving experience for the author of the story as well as for group members. The sharing of intimate material stimulates the process of meaning-making.

Wedding train: A group member wanted to find a way to connect with both her mother and her daughter. She found a photo of her mother in her wedding dress. She then obtained a photo of her daughter in her wedding dress and then of herself in her own wedding dress. She had three copies made of each photo and framed them so that each received a vertical three picture frame: grandmother–mother–daughter, each on their wedding day, in their wedding dresses.

Activity – Like Sand through an Hourglass

Materials: 8 × 10 plastic tray, sand, collection of seashells, rocks, pebbles, small spoon, and a fork for each member.

Description: This is a Zen tray activity. Pour sand into the trays. Provide a variety of shells and the like and supply utensils. Ask the members to relax while the facilitator reads a short passage regarding family/legacy. It is recommended that they listen. Next, create a visual arrangement with their tray by placing items, raking sand with the tools provided.

Ideas for Readings: Short books (*The Missing Piece* and *The Giving Tree* by Shel Silverstein, 2006, 2014); fables available by moral topic: family, relationships, trust, and so on.

Therapeutic Intent: This is a meditative, reflective activity. Engaging in creating a Zen Garden is believed to increase perspective and stimulate creativity.

Activity – Legacy Rap

Materials: Large poster board and colored markers.

Description: This is a group Haiku activity. Begin by defining Haiku as a Japanese poem of 17 syllables. There are three lines; five syllables, seven syllables, and five syllables. The poem depicts images and senses of the natural world. Group members brainstorm a general topic or, if appropriate, the facilitator selects a topic. The members collaborate to create the Haiku. Box 6.1 demonstrates an example of a Haiku.

BOX 6.1   LEGACY RAP

Haiku 1

> Family is great
> Even in-laws make me smile
> Blessings all around.

Haiku 2

> Looking behind me
> I see choices made and not
> A road to my *now*.

Therapeutic Intent: Anyone can create a poem. Facilitators found that members learned the skill quickly and created poems on a whim or when given a specific theme. This is a tried-and-true group activity. Some members reported finding uses for a Haiku outside of the Legacy Group experience that proved therapeutic for them.

Activity – The Third Degree

Materials: Pen, paper, prompts and interview questions.

Description: This is an exercise involving taking and giving an oral history. Members break off into pairs or into groups of three. Offer prompts and/or interview questions having one member interview another. Allow the interviewee to answer at length; explain the power of open-ended and clarifying questions. If answers are given at length, then ideally only one or two questions are asked, and this is the goal. Request that the interviewer take only brief notes during the interaction. Members will switch roles and ask the same questions, or the exercise can be designed to use different questions. After interviewing is complete, each member shares with the other group members what they have learned about their partner.

Therapeutic Intent: Members will learn how to conduct an oral history and how to help the authors expand upon their story. Taking an oral history is a skill that requires active listening and motivational interviewing skills. The one-on-one interview about intimate stories and then sharing what was heard serves to enhance group cohesion.

Activity – Legacy Makes Good Sense

Materials: Items that will stimulate all five senses. Examples: *Sight*: Photos, postcards, old calendars, comic strips, baseball cards, "antique" lunch boxes, or teacups.

Hearing: Wind, waves, dogs barking, birds or crickets, rain falling, children playing, the crack of a bat, or choir music. *Smell*: Essential oils, shampoo, powder, cologne/perfume, or dryer sheets. *Taste*: Offer a plate of cookies to members, pass out lemons, or use small bowls with which to taste various spices. *Touch*: In a bag have various items for members to reach in, touch and feel, without looking (e.g., stuffed toy, matchbox car, a rock, shell, doll house furniture, paintbrush, or glasses). Be creative!

Description: Go through each of the senses. *Sight*: Display a sight item or have the members select from a set of picture cards. Give the group members approximately one minute to reflect on the item. Next, give the group members two minutes to write down their thoughts. *Hearing*: Play one or two recordings and ask the members to write down their experience. *Smell*: Have a common perfume, flower, or something of a common smell for folks. Again, have them write down their thoughts and/or memories. *Taste*: Bring something for members to sample that is a commonly known taste. And again, have the members write down their associations. *Touch*: This is the last sense. Have items for members to touch, possibly soft items. Ask the members to share memories, stories, and associations that arise: what does this remind me of? How was this experience for me? How might it be important to someone else? Go through all five senses before having members share.

Therapeutic Intent: Members are reminded that life experiences and resulting wisdom occurs in all five senses. Some senses are more heavily utilized and relied upon by humans (i.e., sight, hearing), although lived experiences and memories can be tapped from each sense.

Activity – Turning Life's Pages

Materials: Pen, paper, and examples of stationary for finished products.

Description: This is a memoir-writing exercise. Ask the members to imagine their life as if broken into five major chapters. These chapters may be sequential (e.g., childhood, adolescence, adulthood, careers, parenting) or they may also be topic-related (e.g., countries I lived in) or based on values (e.g., the greatest act of kindness, generosity, friendship, faith, and love). What are the chapters you wish to use? Give each chapter a title. Next, offer a summary within each chapter. Then go back and add a few bullet points. Try to add at least three bullet points to each chapter. Next, can you think of the best thing that happened during that "chapter" or the worst? Review your whole document thus far. What would you consider a major turning point? Is it already written there? If not, write it now. Allow any members to share their experience.

Therapeutic Intent: People often equate memoir writing to autobiography, which can be overwhelming. Neither needs to be an overwhelming task. Group members will learn that a memoir may begin with as little as a one-hour group session. It is helpful to point out that this project may be easily continued outside of the group. Members are welcome to bring ongoing projects into group to share.

Activity – Legacy Tunes

Materials: Pens, paper, access to the internet, and one or two apps for searching music or lyrics.

Description: Ask the members to list two to three events from their life. These events could be significant moments (e.g., births, deaths, and marriages), accomplishments, challenges, turning points, crises, celebrations, and the like. Members are then asked to assign a song to each significant moment. Members are encouraged to use a song title, a line from the lyrics, genre, year, and so on. For example, a member may list their wedding day, birth of their son, or a job relocation (Box 6.2). Song assignments may include *Unchained Melody* as that was their first dance; *Bad, Bad Leroy Brown* as his son was named after his grandfather, Leroy; or the song *Dirty Water*, as it references Boston to which he was transferred earlier in his career. Have the members share their lists. An added feature is for the facilitator to locate the music on the internet to play for the group.

BOX 6.2   LEGACY TUNES

My Wedding: Unchained Melody. This was our wedding song. This was our first dance of the night, but to this day when this song plays, I still grab my wife for a quick dance. She thinks that I'm crazy, but really, I think she loves it.

The Birth of My Son: Bad, Bad, Leroy Brown. My son is named Leroy after my father. I have been singing the song to him since he was born. When people asked him his name when he was little, he would respond "Bad, Bad Leroy Brown"; that was cute until he began adding things like "but you can call me 'Sir.' " My wife was not pleased.

Job Transfer: Dirty Water. I don't know any words other than the first line of the chorus, but I always have to belt it out. It references "Boston you're my home" and my job transfer to Boston in my mid-twenties was a great one. So happy I took that chance!

Therapeutic Intent: This exercise sparks creativity with legacy and helps members get in touch with memories. In addition, members are encouraged to experience connections with memories that they had not previously seen. The more connections that are made with memories, the stronger the experience becomes. This activity tends to be a very fun for members. They enjoy searching, pairing the music, and sharing their logic with others.

This activity may be continued outside of the group. A song list of 10–12 could be burned onto a CD and given to someone as a Legacy Gift. Create a list of songs and write a brief explanation regarding choices on the CD cover/insert. Members are welcome to bring ongoing projects into group sessions to share.

Week 10: Last Week of Reflective Processing Exercises

Activity – Exploring and Preserving Food

Materials: Pens, recipe cards, and paper.

Description: Members will recreate a family cookbook. Have group members make a list of recipes they want to include. These recipes can be secret family recipes, cultural favorites (Box 6.3), or simply a list of food they enjoy eating, with whom and where (Box 6.4). Possibly there are stories to go along with them. Request that members bring recipes to group to copy them for their Family Cookbook. Offer the idea that they may include "food stories" that can be told with each recipe. One recipe from each member will be given to the facilitator who will create a *Legacy Group Cookbook* to be handed out at the end of the group experience. You may want to suggest that members can bring a food item to the group for the last group session. Encourage any member bringing food to share about their recipe, its story, how they have been keeper of this meaning, and how they will continue to pass it on.

BOX 6.3 FAVORITE FOODS

Guacamole and chips (with Barry and John during the Pat's game for 27 years running!)

Blueberry pancakes (as often and as many as I can) with whoever I am with.

Brownies (warm, with vanilla ice cream, and hot fudge is a given) with my wife, late night, during a movie when kids are sleeping. Always my favorite date.

BOX 6.4 FAMILY RECIPES

Mom's cinnamon rolls
Uncle Larry's spaghetti sauce
The cranberry sauce (for every Thanksgiving!)
Toll house cookies with a twist

Therapeutic Intent: Members are reminded that important family stories are found at the simplest of places, like the kitchen table. What some members considered a normal part of their day, food, was viewed differently by others. *Doesn't everyone eat breakfast for dinner on Tuesdays? Everyone has spaghetti on their birthday, don't they? I was 14 when someone first served me corn-on-the-cob as a side dish; we ate it as a main course!* Memories give us the opportunity to reflect on "simple" experiences. The group serves to help members find ways to preserve and share these stories with future generations.

Family food: A group member shared nostalgia about Doo Dads (i.e., Chex Mix) in her family. Her paternal grandmother had the secret recipe that included X will not break confidentiality! But know this, she brought in a batch, it was so good and indeed sparked debate about the variety of bits that make a mix special versus the purity of the True Chex. Good times (great mix!).

Therapeutic legacy activities in Phase II assist in transitioning members from a place of unfamiliarity and little-known expectations to a trusting and supporting place in which deeply explorative and meaningful legacy work can be pursued. Members engage in both rapport-building and reflecting exercises that allow each to experience their own space and at a comfortable pace to work on activity-based legacy projects. At this juncture of the group experience they have worked together, laughed, eaten food, made music and poems. They have shared challenges and cried together. Clearly, each group creates its own legacy. Over the next two sessions, the facilitator will guide members with the task of celebrating the group legacy and identifying members' next steps.

Phase III: Process the Group Experience and Consider Future Plans

As the group cycle ends, members may have mixed feelings. Some may express sadness to end the experience, while others may express their gratefulness to have been a part of it. Facilitators use these last two sessions to assist members in processing these feelings and their overall experience. Many members may also have questions regarding ongoing legacy work: What are the next steps and how can they address their future plans?

Week 11: Transitioning to Termination

Activity – Pen Pal from the Past

Materials: Pen, paper, and stationary.

Description: Explain to the group members that they will write or begin to write a letter. The letter is addressed to someone specific (i.e., a child, favorite niece, sibling, special neighborhood child, or unborn grandchild) or to no one in particular. Remind members that they may choose the topic and person to whom the letter will be addressed and written to. Allow a few minutes of writing time. Giving a prompt when there are two minutes remaining will allow the group members time to wrap things up.

Therapeutic Intent: This exercise allows members to have an intimate experience with a significant person from their past. Writing one letter may prompt more letters to the same person or perhaps new letters to different people. Whatever the result, members will likely process and pair many events and people in their life story, some of which may now be shared and passed on.

Letter box: An older adult member (aged 70+ years) hoped to leave something for his grandchildren. He committed to writing each grandchild a letter, one per month, sealing it and placing it away in a box. The letter contained writings ranging from his thoughts about current events to the price of milk and bread. He would share what was playing in the movies and who were the big music or TV stars. Each grandchild would receive their box, their own piece of their grandfather when they turned 18 years old.

Week 12: A Time to Celebrate and Final Reflections

Activity – Making Note of Your Legacy

Materials: Paper and pen.

Description: *Legacy Group* closes as it began, with the opportunity to reflect using a brief, albeit different, writing prompt. Group members are told that they will be given a prompt to which they will write for five minutes. It is important not to overthink, but, instead, "free write." Request that they write continuously for the allotted time even if they believe that they have finished.

Prompt: After participating in this 12-week *Legacy Group* experience, describe your understanding and experience of family. Has your understanding and experience of family changed since you began this process? What is your legacy and how will you share it? How do you see yourself as keeper of the meaning? It is helpful to offer a two-minute warning before time is up. Allow any member who wants to share their thoughts the time to do so.

Therapeutic Intent: Members have completed 12 sessions consisting of activities and processing with other older adults on a similar journey. It is likely and hopeful that their concept of legacy, family, and "keeper of the meaning" has deepened, and this writing exercise offers them a time and place to reflect upon their legacy.

Last, pass out the *Legacy Group Cookbooks*. This has become a popular way to terminate the group experience. Members will have these cookbooks to remind them of this group and how they explored their legacy.

People avoid looking back for many reasons. The cultural language and messages are clear: focus on the future, drive ahead, truck on, face forward. Some individuals struggle with the past due to what they consider poor choices, regrets, or great personal loss. This can result in a debilitating grief that leads to a sense of loss of control and helplessness. However, it has been suggested that taking steps toward remembering is, in fact, taking steps toward healing. Proactively seeking out thoughts and memories can lead to individual empowerment, which is a key to a full and happy life (Gilbert et al., 2020). Similarly, legacy exploration and telling one's story is a proactive way to increase personal empowerment and stimulate a full and happy life. Sharing yourself, your history, and your experiences, whether through journaling, poetry, interviews, or artifacts, are all representations of the person. As an individual may enjoy researching the legacy of a loved one, so too, will someone enjoy researching yours. What will you leave them to find?

Additional Activities for *Activity-Based Legacy Groups*

Activity – The Sum of the Parts

Materials: Poster board; magazines and photos; glue/tape; scissors; and internet access for printing pictures, news headings, and the like.

Description: This is a collage-making activity. Members may bring in their own pictures or they can be supplied. Group members will make a collage by adhering pictures, words, and the like to their poster in random or specific order. Collages may be representative of a specific time, their whole life, or a single event. Members are asked to share their collage and overall theme with the group. Frame for safe keeping.

Therapeutic Intent: A visual and biographical representation may foster a greater understanding of one's interests, values, and place in the story. Hanging up a visual representation allows members to connect with that image and associated thoughts and feelings on a regular basis. This activity allows one to share personal material with the group.

Activity – Treasure Chest for the Ages

Materials: Box to decorate (e.g., shoe box, old shipping box, empty tissue box), craft paper, stickers, contact paper, paintbrush/sponge, and scissors. Mod Podge is a common product used in crafting projects.

Description: Decoupage box. Members will decorate a box as a keepsake with items supplied or with personal photos and pictures from magazines brought in by a group member to use. Fabrics can also be adhered using Mod Podge. The purpose of the box is to store artifacts and memorabilia.

Therapeutic Intent: A decoupage box is a way to keep a variety of legacy items safe that one wishes to pass along in the future (e.g., letters, tickets, playbills). Facilitators may want members to share their experience of making their box, what significance are their decorations, share how it will be used (i.e., to store letters, photos, mementos of events, relationships).

Activity – Making "Note" of Your Legacy

Materials: Pen and paper.

Description: This activity requires journaling without a prompt. Group members are asked to keep a journal throughout the group experience. The opportunity to write in one's journal is given at the start of, or at the end, each group session. Journaling may entail what happens week to week in the group, about what has happened in the member's life over the past week, or random thoughts that they wish to record in their journal, or possibly what is happening in the world. These journal entries may be shared or kept private, depending on how the facilitator and group members wish to use this journaling.

Therapeutic Intent: Members are given few expectations and a great amount of freedom with this activity. They are given the opportunity to write during group. As a result, many members may continue to journal on their own outside of the group.

Activity – Three-Dimensional Lives

Materials: A Shadow Box that can be purchased from a craft store, adhesive and a glue gun, and items to display. These items may include jewelry, eye wear, photos, handkerchiefs, gloves, a pipe, lighter, coins, IDs, sewing needles/thread, knives, baseball, or recipe cards.

Description: Group members are advised to consider a wide variety of items that represent the whole person, a part of the person, or even a moment in time. Items are placed in the shadow box and adhered to the back of box then covered with plexiglass that protects and preserves the displayed items.

Therapeutic Intent: Group members are afforded the opportunity to see how even just a few small items pack a large legacy punch. This is a very artistic, thumbnail representation of one's own life or about a loved one's story.

Activity – A Picture Is Worth a Thousand Stories

Materials: Photo album, pictures, adhesives, and scissors.

Description: Group members place photos into the album in any order. Some may wish to label the photos and sort them in an organized, time-line fashion. Others may choose to make multiple collages throughout their album.

Therapeutic Intent: This activity is carried out with members who have access to family photos. It is a fun way to take on what may be a seemingly overwhelming task; one picture at a time. Members are encouraged to engage in the process by sharing the stories of the photos they included in the album. The process of sorting photos often sparks new memories as well as reinforcing older memories.

Activity – To Rhyme or Not to Rhyme

Materials: Pen, paper; easel paper; and markers, if completed as a group activity.

Description: The Cinquain is a form of a poem that is less intimidating than "writing a poem," as there is no rhyming required. Members are asked to follow the 2–4–6–8–2 structure shown in the example in Box 6.5. The facilitator may offer a completed Cinquain as an example, before asking the group to write a poem together. Potential themes to use are childhood, parenting, history, memories, or legacy.

BOX 6.5 EXAMPLE OF A CINQUAIN POEM

Legacy
by Victoria L. Bacon
One's Roots . . .
People . . . Stories,
Places, history, time,
Engaging in self-reflection,
My roots.

Therapeutic Intent: The Cinquain poem offers members a way to be creative using a different writing style. This has been a popular activity with group members. They seem to enjoy the process and end up writing more Cinquain poems outside of the group.

Activity – Leafing through a Legacy

Materials: Scrapbook or photo album, adhesive, scissors, photos, postcards, letters, notes, flyers, newspaper clippings, articles, awards and certificates, concert, sports, theater tickets, playbills, and the like.

Description: Group members place items into a photo album in any order they wish. Some may wish to label pages and lay them in an organized, time-line fashion. Others may choose to make multiple collages throughout their album.

Therapeutic Intent: Like a photo album, this activity encourages members to enjoy the process of reflecting on their legacy. A scrapbook is a long and committed project; however, it should also be one that is pleasurable. Members are reminded that sharing the stories of completed pages will help stimulate the work of others.

Activity – Planting the Seeds

Materials: Internet access, account login for one genealogical website, the name of a family member with which a participant would like to begin searching and any information available (e.g., full name, birth/death, marriage, career information, place of residence, or children/parent). Please note that Family Search is a free service.

Description: Group members will be encouraged to use one or more websites to begin their initial search. The facilitator may provide a lesson about the best ways to conduct a search and provide worksheets for members to use while searching their family history. It is helpful for members to share strategies used, what was successful, and what they found. A field trip might be considered to a local historical society or invite a speaker to the group experience to review how to research family history.

Therapeutic Intent: This activity affords members interested in conducting research on their genealogy an opportunity to begin that type of exploration. Although some people become focused on researching dates and names, researching genealogy is much more. For instance, newspaper articles shed light on the time period and context. Census records provide information about cultural heritage, places worked, and household members. Church records are a valuable source for births, marriages, and deaths.

Activity – The Proust Phenomenon

Materials: Pen, paper, items to stimulate taste and smell, and The Cookie excerpt by Proust.

Description: A similar activity as the Making Sense of Legacy offers the opportunity to tap into the senses. This activity focuses on two senses: taste and smell. The facilitator explains that we primarily rely on sight and auditory information. Research suggests that odors can cue vivid autobiographical memory, or what is known as the Proust Phenomenon. Further, smells trigger greater emotional responses associated with those memories, compared to other sensory cues. This is because scent and taste information does not get processed in the thalamus, the brain's relay station, but instead goes directly to the limbic system, the brain's emotional center (Jerome, 2019). Offer members a variety of items to smell and taste (e.g., cookies, spices, breads, tea) and have them share the different memories experienced. All activities can be considered an opportunity for brief writing as well.

Therapeutic Intent: This activity provides an opportunity for members to experience memories. Members often report that over the next few days they experienced an increase in awareness around smell and taste.

References

Gilbert, S. J., Bird, A., Carpenter, J. M., Fleming, S. M., Sachdeva, C., & Tsai, P. (2020). Optimal use of reminders: Metacognition, effort, and cognitive offloading. *Journal of Experimental Psychology, 149*(3), 501–517.

Jerome, R. (2019). The time-bending magic of smell. In *Time: The science of memory, the story of our lives*. Meredith Corporation.

Silverstein, S. (2006). *The missing piece*. HarperCollins.

Silverstein, S. (2014). *The giving tree*. HarperCollins.

7

CLINICAL REFLECTIONS

As authors, we had the opportunity to facilitate Legacy Groups in a variety of settings and like any group, each took on an energy and life of its own. Whether group membership consisted of women veterans, community-dwelling older adults, or residents in skilled nursing facilities, various familial and social microcosms blossomed. We followed the Legacy Group curricula reviewed in Chapters 5 and 6, yet unique themes and considerations presented themselves. The following examples and insights into selected demographics are from of our Legacy Group experiences. They offer an exclusively personal glimpse into some special groups of people that an encyclopedia full of methods and data can simply not provide. Each section highlights facilitator reflections involving three different populations: *Women Who Served*, *Adults in Search of Meaning*, and *Older Adults on a Journey*.

Women Who Served

When we began searching for women veterans to participate in a Legacy Group experience, we began with the question: What defines a veteran? In our search for an answer, we learned that the parameters set by the Veterans Administration (VA) includes a variety of factors: years of service, type of duty, and type of discharge, to name a few. Further, veteran status is what allows access to the VA healthcare network as well as to a variety of educational and vocational opportunities. We also learned that a person may have served many years and did not receive an honorable discharge, thus negating their access to veteran status and VA benefits (Szymendra, 2016).

The initial research grant was funded for Legacy Group experiences exclusively for women veterans, as the research team considered them to be an

DOI: 10.4324/9781003298168-9

underserved veteran population. Women veterans self-report a severe shortage of female-specific programs in general, but specifically regarding military sexual trauma and for alcohol and drug treatment. After giving years of dedicated service to their country, many are left feeling alienated by the organization that was created to assist them (Cassidy, 2017). We posited that women veterans would appreciate, and benefit from, the opportunity to engage in legacy exploration in a wellness group setting along with other women who had similar military experiences. What we found was that women veterans were eager to participate in a group that connected them with other women veterans. For many of these women, a Legacy Group spoke to their needs.

Pre-Group Screening Reflections

Screening was an essential tool that provided us with baseline information. Having a homogeneous group of women veterans resulted in members quickly feeling safe and supported by their peers. Screening involved identifying veteran status, and a full set of additional veteran-specific demographics, including branch of service, length of service, combat experiences, age of enlistment and discharge, and psychological and/or physical disabilities. We noted that group members could share rich and transformative experiences whether we selected members with varied demographics or by strategically narrowing the selection criteria by including only combat veterans, or members from a specific time/period/war, or even gender-based groups. Overall, intentionality in selection was the key. What we found was, women veterans, in their desire to connect with other like-minded women, who served their country, appreciated the opportunity to engage in another mission together. They brought their personal attributes and strengths as well as their military skills with them: a desire to support, to assist, and to never leave another behind. As facilitators, we learned that separating the personal woman from the military woman was no easy task. Clearly, these women were called to serve as a direct result of their personal attributes and now the two parts of their lives became one.

As we interviewed women veterans for the Legacy Group experience, we were consistently impressed with their openness to share specific military credentials, including length of service, duty assignments, and discharge information. Some of the women were honorably discharged at the end of their enlistment; some were retired after many years of service, while others were honorably discharged or retired due to injury or disability. These women had been assigned to various bases across the United States, Europe, and to war zones in the Middle East. Duties ranged from military police work, guarding prisoners, to convoy truck drivers in Afghanistan and Iraq. Others were equipped for tank and large truck mechanics, accounting assignments in large Air Force bases, as well as supervision of troops in hot spots where split-second decisions were pivotal for troop safety. We noted immense pride as these women spoke of their dedication to duty, and the honor they felt having served their country. We also sensed their eagerness to begin the group experience. It became increasingly clear that there was a loss of connection with other women veterans since their return to civilian life. We were told by many that, after discharge, they returned home to their civilian life as wife, mother, sister, daughter, employee, or student and sometimes all these roles. They found little time and few opportunities to seek out and connect with other women veterans.

On one occasion, we conducted a screening with a woman veteran who was particularly anxious about the legacy exploration and preservation. She was intrigued, but clearly stated that she felt unable to identify her legacy and therefore any worthwhile preservation project. We placed her into a Legacy Group based on the potential support we believed that she would receive. As hoped and suspected, the vitality of personalities and the variety of military experiences in group created a balance that offered just enough familiarity for safety, and more than enough novelty for legacy exploration. Although reluctant at first to accept help with what she perceived as her job, as the group evolved, she gratefully accepted support from group members and thrived in the Legacy Group due to *cohesion* and support. Further, she later shared that since returning to civilian life, she had been the financial, emotional, and even physical backbone of her family. Particularly after her husband left, she was the sole provider and fixer of all things ranging from broken toasters to broken hearts. She did not have time to take her own emotional roll call. However, the insight she gained during the group experience regarding her own needs led her to acknowledge a sense of loss over the past few years. Her experience was *cathartic* and a direct result of her brave willingness to accept the support and feedback of her fellow women veterans. This is just one of the many occurrences where we observed the transformative power of the group dynamic at such an individual level.

Screening members for a Legacy Group is an important time to identify special needs and/or learning differences that may impact individual functioning in a group setting. The women veterans we interviewed were diverse in educational level and overall cognitive functioning. It appeared that some member differences in functioning may be due to performance anxiety, an emotional challenge, or possibly residual effects from head trauma or another service-related injury or issue. These differences were not always evident in screenings yet were addressed as they arose by making modifications to directions and exercises to suit each member's understanding and ability.

As the following example suggests, some special needs were clearly articulated by the group members. On one occasion, a potential group member let it be known that she would require seating against a wall that offered her full view of exits. She proceeded to educate us on the importance of this consideration for all veterans. The type of chair was also a predetermining factor required for her to attend. She then offered a list of reasons why this should be an important consideration for all veterans. In all seriousness, she did require some degree of cushioning and support for comfort due to chronic pain because of a service injury. Fortunately, our research had prepared us for these requested needs; the former more commonly made by combat or trauma veterans, but the latter made by many veterans experiencing disability and chronic pain. As a result, we tried to select meeting rooms based not only on privacy but on comfort as well. Soft chairs with high backs were favored around a meeting table that provided space between group members and offered the ability to spread materials out freely. Please imagine, if you can, this member's response when we were invited to conduct the group experience in the spacious boardroom of a local university. Tall-backed, leather chairs that adjusted in every imaginable direction and an oak conference table that stretched into eternity. We were even greeted by a university executive who encouraged the women to help themselves to the coffee and cold drinks from his personal kitchen. This woman veteran may have found a seat with a view of an exit, but she decided not to use it, as she quickly became immersed in the welcome that whispered safe and comfortable.

Phase I: Supportive Group Environment and Realistic Goal Setting (Weeks 1–3)

We found the early weeks took on an energy and life of its own. The women had been so depleted of connection with their sisters that our early tasks were geared toward gently guiding the group to accomplish the necessary business of the first few sessions. For example, sharing contact information is always recommended in case of illness or schedule changes. Yet these women began swapping their information almost immediately upon entering the group room. They were quick to share their own information, as well as tips on navigating the VA Healthcare system, and how to seek out assistance for disability or employment applications.

These initial weeks were also an important time to identify what accommodations and modifications were needed that had not presented during the screening process. For instance, we noted the importance of lighting in the room; strong light was important for many to be able to read, but we were mindful to avoid glare as light sensitivity was problematic for others. When any type of projection was used, we found that checking in with each member about comfort and visual clarity was particularly important. We suspected that some could not see well on occasion, but they said nothing of it as they were simply glad to have been asked. We made sure that general housekeeping items were repeated weekly to ensure members' ease of access to restrooms, drinking fountains, and seating.

We were afforded the opportunity to witness the sharing of a wide range of early legacy project ideas. Some women came to the table with multiple ideas for exploring their legacy or creating a legacy project, whereas others were overwhelmed, not knowing where to begin. We would often remind them that any legacy idea can be fulfilling, big or small. Although encouragement from facilitators was appreciated, the women veterans clearly responded to the reassurance offered by their peers.

Consider a woman veteran who had returned to civilian life after retiring from a 25-year military career, where she had been in charge of soldiers who provided materials for troops in war zones. She has been honored not only for her ability to lead and for her organizational skills but also for her dedication and duty. Yet as a civilian, she was a wife and mother. She shared that she did not believe that her military service was acknowledged, appreciated, or could ever be fully understood by her family. She felt angry and hurt. As a result, she planned to create an extensive scrapbook about her military career that she did not intend to share with her family. She informed us that she planned to put it away so it would be discovered after she died. Her fellow veterans, with great sensitivity and kindness, validated her feelings by sharing their own disappointment about returning to civilian life. They also shared how they were able to move past their anger and hurt; some women were still in the process of working on these pieces.

Other women veterans shared stories about coming to the realization that their children were not acting selfish or cruel but were just being children and thinking and seeing through children's eyes. Over time, this group member was able to internalize feedback from her peers and adopt a new perspective. Through careful and sensitive process, *corrective recapitulation of primary family group*, she was able to find new ways to relate to family members. She eventually decided to create a smaller scrapbook, a legacy project that she would design with her youngest child. The *altruism* of these women veterans was profound as they *imparted information* to one another. Each week we witnessed increased *cohesion* and the transformative power of the group experience. Imagine a family member finding the legacy project as first proposed, one created from a place of anger and pain, and left behind out of spite. Instead, her legacy came from a place of love and forgiveness, for herself and others; it served to create connection and to share a personal legacy with future generations.

Phase II: Personal Legacy Work; Guidance and Support (Weeks 4–10)

As the weeks progressed, we observed an increase in *cohesion* among the women. Attendance was remarkably consistent, and members would become concerned if someone did not show up or let the facilitators know that they would be absent. The woman veterans, true to their training, were always eager to hear how another member's legacy project was progressing, sharing where they had found certain materials or where they had wartime photos copied. Trusting others, even other women veterans, is not always an easy task for this population. However, throughout the group experience, we witnessed that these women take risks, reach out, and share their memories, often with extremely sensitive personal material. As such, when a trusted source outside of the group was identified (i.e., locating comrades, restoring wartime photos), their contact information was shared liberally. Sometimes, however, that trusted source was inside the group.

During a session one group member chose to bring in photographs and share her wartime experiences when she served in Iraq. As she delved more deeply, her head lowered, her voice softened and slowed. She was visibly struggling to go on. After a few quiet moments, faint whispers could be heard as we noted another woman veteran, seated close by, had begun to offer soft, encouraging comments regarding her own service in the Middle East, suggesting that she had seen and experienced similar situations. The original speaker slowly raised her head and completed her story for the group, yet her eyes never left her group-time hero as if drawing the strength necessary from them to complete her mission. Other members were riveted by the story, remaining silent throughout. Upon completion, all the women veterans sat in a respectful silence, offering no comments until she asked for feedback directly.

Over time, we observed many tendencies of the women veterans that were unique. This population of women who enlisted to serve their country and took an oath to that promise. We witnessed teamwork, the ability to lead, and punctuality. They were trained to precisely follow time schedules. Arriving at the appointed time is considered being late. Therefore, we learned to arrive early to *Women Who Served* Legacy Groups as they were usually there 10–15 minutes before us and at the table with their materials out, arranged, and ready! Although these group members leaned toward precision, as facilitators, it was important to instill a sense of flexibility. Oftentimes members needed to attend necessary medical or psychological appointments and felt uncomfortable asking to leave early or arrive late. The result was a culture in which the women felt safe to truly engage, and we fully enjoyed the *universally* respectful nature in which these women veterans interacted during the group experience.

Let it be known that they enjoyed engaging with one another in playful banter. If not careful, their excited conversations would sufficiently derail any planned sessions. On one occasion, the women began to reminisce about some challenging and unpleasant assignments that they were required to complete on base after returning from a long and dangerous convoy mission: cleaning the latrines. As they shared memories of those sights and smells, their language became more punctuated, and their word choice was as foul, loud, and deep as what they described. They had eased back into utilizing profanity that was likely the typical vernacular of wartime military. Fortunately, veterans fall back easily and, as such, these excited exchanges needed only to be gently curtailed to proceed with the group process.

As the weeks went on, we had the pleasure of observing the drive to complete a mission that was very strong for each member. Some women became laser-focused, while others became more distressed about not reaching a specific project goal. We found it necessary to remind them that they can continue with their legacy journey at a comfortable pace, that a project in-process should be considered a success based on their personally set goals. Group members offered suggestions with how to complete a smaller piece of the exploration or preservation work that could segue to a larger legacy project.

One member who had spent her career in the Air Force had recently retired and returned to live in her childhood home and care for her mother who was diagnosed with dementia. In their walks around the neighborhood, this veteran would reminisce with her mother about who had lived in the various houses when she was growing up. She remembered neighbors who were kind to them as children in the neighborhood and the store that they would go to for penny candy or something cold on a hot summer day. She decided to take photos of these houses and former stores, write brief memories of each, check in with some older neighbors who still lived in their homes to collect accurate names and facts, create a photo book, and had photo books printed. She planned to keep one and review the memories with her mother periodically and give books to the neighbors who helped her identify and preserve these special memories.

Her fellow group member's favorite photo was a nondescript building that was presently an apartment house but had once been a small corner store with an apartment above where the owners lived. This woman veteran shared her memories of riding bikes on hot summer days and stopping at this store. Although there was no air conditioning, the store felt cool, and the owner always welcomed them with a smile. The children pooled their coins and would buy popsicles to share. After paying, they would gather outside at the corner of the store and split the frozen pops against the building's corner. She shared that it was the perfect way to be sure that the popsicles split equally. Her memories were delightful and poignant, making the group experience even richer. This member was so moved by the feedback and compliments that she received from others that she began to reach out to the people from her old neighborhood asking them if they had contact information for anyone who had lived in the close-knit community of her childhood. Her plan was to connect with those whose contact information was found and to give a copy of the photo book to them as well. She envisioned a contact list in which past neighbors could reconnect if they desired. Her legacy project transformed from one that she created for herself and used to connect with her mother into one that she would share with the people from her childhood neighborhood. This is a wonderful example of a smaller legacy project evolving organically into a larger and far-reaching community legacy. Please, be mindful, not all veteran-status members are able to make such adjustments. Some remained in military mode, hyper focused, and struggled with the concept of unfinished business. Fortunately, most were able to make shifts and embrace the freedom that is inherent in an ongoing legacy journey.

Consider the shift made by the women veteran who was initially angry and hurt upon returning to her family. She wanted her service to be acknowledged. Her children wanted Mom. Participating in a Legacy Group provided the opportunity for her to work through some of her feelings. This allowed her to create a photo album in tandem with her youngest daughter. They both agreed that the binder would be placed on the elder daughter's bed for her to find during her first night away at college. We witnessed how the trajectory of a person's emotions can become gently altered by the facilitators and enhanced and fostered by the other members of the group. This woman veteran received validation and support from her peers and, as a result, retooled her plans for the preservation of her legacy project.

Phase III: Reflection and Celebration (Weeks 11 and 12)

During the final two weeks, we guided these women in a series of reflective activities. Many of them commented on how they enjoyed reconnecting with other women veterans. Others were grateful for the opportunity to share important, although sometimes difficult, memories that they had not discussed or even remembered for many years. One member shared how thankful she was for her Legacy Group experience, as it offered her the support and guidance that she needed to open boxes of photos from her Middle East deployment that she had stored in the back of a closet since her discharge. Initially, she believed that she had simply become too busy reentering civilian life. As time went on, she continued to fill her time with new civilian-life business and, at least part consciously, suppressed her wartime memories. Further, the longer the photos remained packed away, the more reluctant she became to open the boxes. She informed her sisters-in-arms that because they had shared similar experiences and spoke of them freely, including their reluctance to do so, that she had decided to open the box and access these photos for her legacy project. Although she admitted to shedding tears while looking through them, she also reflected on the new perspectives in which she was able to view them.

Consider as well, the veteran discussed previously, who was hurt and angry as to how her own family appeared to disregard her military service. Her initial I'll show them project, transformed into a mother–daughter project that stimulated connection and more specifically, conversation regarding events that occurred while serving in the military. During the last weeks, she reflected on the project's impact on her, her daughter, and their relationship. As a result of her reflection, she informed us that when she dropped her older daughter off at college in the fall, she would leave the photos album hidden under the pillow for her to find her first night away from home. She was certain that her daughter would be comforted not only by the pictures but by the artwork on each page created by her other daughter during her legacy work.

Reflecting on process and individual goals are an important part of closing a Legacy Group experience. Yet, so too, is celebrating! We used the second half of the final session to showcase projects: bringing snacks/drinks and closing with the same journal prompt we opened with and comparing them. Celebrating took many different forms. For our last group session, everyone agreed to bring something to snack on. We had planned on conducting an activity and then enjoying some downtime with light conversation and food for the last 20 minutes. This may have been too broad of a description for the evening. One woman arrived to the group that night with two bottles of wine and a filet of salmon the length of your arm. We had no kitchen or tools and were uncomfortable about the wine as this group was hosted in a local rectory. As we silently wondered together which issue to deal with first, the answer came literally bounding through the door. One veteran had brought her giant, yellow Labrador retriever whom she had decorated with red bows and sleigh bells. Celebrations became a bit more defined, but no less enjoyable. We celebrated goals, perseverance, and success; we celebrated unity and individuals; we celebrated freedom and family; mostly though, we celebrated each other.

The veterans we worked with bonded with one another through their pride in serving their country and in their minority status, as women, both in the military and in their civilian lives. By the end of the *Women Who served* Legacy Group, another sisterhood had evolved. And it was clear that this time connections and opportunities for support would not be lost. They truly would not leave a sister behind.

Adults in Search of Meaning

In 2013–2014, we broadened the group membership criteria. Newly received funding did not restrict outreach to women veterans. As such, the research and community service project was extended to older adults living in the community, regardless of veteran status, who expressed interest in exploring and preserving their legacy. Many answered the call. We began offering Legacy Groups at Councils on Aging, in a university setting, with residents in assisted-living and skilled nursing facilities. Fortunately, we were both prepared and excited. We wish to share the reflections about *Adults in Search of Meaning* Legacy Groups, adults living in the community.

Pre-Group Screening Reflections

As we screened for eligibility for *Adults in Search of Meaning* Legacy Groups, we were faced with centuries of deeply engrained cultural history. For many, this history directly influenced their motivation for legacy exploration. For others, the influence was subtle but equally important to their quest. Older adults were joining a Legacy Group for several reasons: to leave something behind, to create something for a special person, or to seek answers to specific questions. Yet there were also similarities in their motivations and goals. Certain life events had been experienced by these members. As a result, these generational cohorts' events helped connect one another in ways that even they did not fully understand at the time (i.e., lived experiences, world events). Every potential member we spoke with had a desire to reach back and dust off a memory and tell their story. They each felt a need to share the wisdom of their own experience and to create something that would outlast their time in this life.

As facilitators, we observed that, like other Legacy Group experiences (i.e., women veterans), older adults presented with challenges – physical and cognitive challenges that needed accommodations. Difficulty with ambulation, balance, and fine motor skills were common, as were visual and auditory considerations. Short- and long-term memories, processing speed, and verbal comprehension and expression were challenges that surfaced regularly. Clearly, living independently did not mean living without hurdles, yet group members' attendance and commitment to the Legacy Group suggested that they had the desire and ability to explore, persevere, as well as connect.

Phase I: Supportive Group Environment and Realistic Goal Setting (Weeks 1–3)

A safe and supportive environment is critical throughout the group process and is established early using brief activities. Sometimes, the group offers you a golden nugget. For example, one man had walked the outside running track before coming to the first session of group. Upon learning this, each week the members would call out to him as he entered the room asking him if he had walked the track today, and if so, for what distance? He enjoyed his flash of celebrity each week, and the other members were equally entertained by this banter. The banter was used to include all members, as they offered remarks and connected with one another – a great way to get into the here and now. Group members benefited from an overall increase in *cohesion*.

Good old-fashioned icebreakers served this function as well. During one exercise in which group members were instructed to journal about family, one member appeared anxious. She stated that her schooling had been subpar, and she was clearly self-conscious about her writing. We reminded her that writing and/or sharing was optional and that she could express herself in any way she selected: narrative, words, drawings, or concepts. She began to write with great concentration. Group members then had the opportunity to share their writing. The woman who appeared anxious about engaging in a writing exercise was first to offer to read her journal entry. She had written in phrases about getting a big meal ready and calling her children to the table. She recalled how she would provide reminders to wash hands, move chairs, and bring serving dishes to the table. It was clear that she was proud of those mealtime memories and the delicious food that she cooked for her children, even with the challenges of a limited single-parent income. When she finished, the group was initially silent, in awe of what she had written. Some thought it sounded like the beginning of a book. Others believed it sounded like poetry. Before: anxious, less educated, self-conscious;

after: author and poet. This *Older Adult in Search of Meaning* Legacy Group experience, elevated by the genuine respect and support offered by her peers, led to group *cohesiveness*.

Creating legacy projects is exciting and daunting for older adults. The sheer number of years lived brought some unexpected stories and experiences to the table, potentially referencing 100–150 years from the past. One of our oldest group members shared the story of her father who had been a slave in the South when he was young. Although freed years before her birth, she was certain that his experiences left an indelible impact upon him and the way he raised his children. Unsure about how to honor his legacy, she believed that her father raised honest, kind, and proud individuals in the face of adversity.

Phase II: Personal Legacy Work; Guidance and Support (Weeks 4–10)

Each week, group members shared, *imparting information*, their own memories and stories and offered feedback to others. They learned from one another about big things like different worldviews, as well as small things like volunteering opportunities. One older woman volunteered with a program that linked local high school students with older adults for conversation and connection. She informed us that she needed to leave promptly each week to meet with her high school student. At the close of each session, she proudly pulled out her scheduler and shared what she and her young high school friend had planned for the day. Some of their outings included participating in a clothing drive, collecting used books for a book sale, or simply seating and talking over coffee about what was happening in their lives. Other group members were intrigued not only with the activities but also with the obvious importance of this program and they admired her commitment.

Another wonderful example from the *Adults in Search of Meaning* Legacy Group conducted in a highly concentrated Portuguese area was that many members were immigrants or first-generation US citizens. The *universality* was observed in their shared experiences and memories. Dedication to family and food were common bonds among this community. Conversations were typically quite animated as group members spoke of memories of certain foods and shared how their mother or grandmother replaced ingredients that were scarce or too costly with others. They talked of how recipes have been passed down for generations, many with nonspecific measurements such as a pinch of that or a teacup of that. Solutions to problems were eagerly shared. This *universality* was observed in other ways as well. Members connected through memories of the Great Depression Era cooking, and World War II events, including women joining the workforce. They recalled early school days in one-room schoolhouses, girls wanting to go to college but finances and/or families that believed to educate only the boys, sewing clothes for their family, and caring for older relatives until they passed.

Each rich and poignant glimpse of a time melted into history served as beautiful reminders, connecting stories, and potential legacy projects.

We were not always looking back. Many of the group members used current technologies and incorporated them into their legacy work (e.g., printing and repairing pictures, researching, and creating family trees). One older woman shared that she did not have a computer and as such was unable to complete the desired searches. Another member explained that the Council on Aging had computers and printers that were accessible, and that she would be happy to help her learn some basic computer skills to search topics of interest. Each week they arrived deep in conversation about a computer-related issue and continued to sit next to each other as their friendship grew. This initial act of *altruism*, in offering her time and knowledge, of course benefited them and as a result benefited the group.

When we were looking back, there were always members who struggled to find legacy artifacts until it was pointed out to them by another group member. Sometimes the pointing out required some heavy convincing. For example, we suggested that group members bring a small item to the next session and provide a brief explanation of its connection to their personal legacy. One woman shared that she didn't have many memorabilia as she had moved into a very small apartment. At the next meeting, she arrived with a large brown bag which she preceded to place conspicuously on the table. She was often solemn, more serious than other members, and was convinced to join a Legacy Group by her friend: "it will be good for you," so this big old, crumpled paper bag caught the group's attention. Then she uncharacteristically offered to begin during the sharing portion of the session. Out of the bag, she pulled a toddler-sized red velvet dress. She had originally made it for her daughter. The dress had been passed down and worn by three generations of little girls over the holidays. She showed us different photographs in which her daughter, granddaughter, and great granddaughter were each wearing this handmade dress during Christmas holiday events. She was saving the dress, hoping to see yet one more generation wear it. She was caught a bit off guard by the reaction of group members and all the comments about her sewing skills were unwarranted. Group members offered feedback about next steps: write about the dress-making process; include any patterns that would be helpful; include photos and place the dress in a shadow box that might become the focal piece in her apartment. Sometimes what is so clearly wondrous and amazing to others is masked in normalcy, as such, takes the mystery and romance of generations of red velvet dresses for granted.

As in any group experience, the journey is often more important than the actual completion of the end goal (i.e., legacy project). Consider our group member who had recently retired from a prestigious executive position in a large company. She presented as very professional, her clothing and manner suited for any high-intensity boardroom meeting. She was focused on making decisions about her legacy project and completing it efficiently. Her plan was to organize the boxes (and boxes and boxes) of photographs for both her own and her husband's families. If she didn't recognize the person in the photo, it was discarded. Efficient! As the group experience progressed and she engaged in various legacy exercises, her perspective began to shift. She considered a smaller, more attainable goal; one that allowed her to spend time with the actual photos. During one session, she shared that she had come across a photo of her husband when he was a small boy seated on his father's shoulders. As she continued to sort through them, she again came across a father with a son upon his shoulders; however, this photo was of her son and her husband. Then her legacy lightbulb went off! She located a recent photo of her son and her grandson on his shoulders. The three-photo matted frame is now mounted in a vertical format and hanging in their home. An achievable outcome: a short-term project that began her journey by looking through generations of photographs with an appreciation for ideas that could produce satisfying artifacts and the opportunity for meaning-making.

Phase III: Reflection and Celebration (Weeks 11 and 12)

Sometimes legacy projects have clearly defined boundaries and edges. Scrapbooks and journals can be seen and touched. But at other times, legacy projects sneak up on you and are more difficult to describe and yet facilitate growth and connection. One of the *Adults in Search of Meaning* Legacy Groups was made up of women professionals who met weekly during lunch. One of the group members decided to create a time capsule with her grandson. They began collecting artifacts of interest: coins dated with their year of birth, favorite magazines, a CD of their favorite music artists. During the second to last session, she announced that she and her grandson had decided to host an extended family gathering. Each person was to bring a favorite dish and one artifact for the time capsule. The legacy gift was the family time capsule event. Future generations will enjoy the time capsule memorabilia.

Older Adults on a Journey

Once we secured funding and where we were able to expand our outreach into the community, we offered Legacy Groups to older adults in assisted-living and long-term care facilities. Although previous screenings were conducted individually, a group screening was offered in these settings, as we believed that this format would provide us with sufficient information about cognitive and physical abilities, as well as interest and motivation for joining a Legacy Group. We worked directly with the Activities Director to arrange a time, day, and length of session that best suited the needs of the residents. Conducting Legacy Groups in these settings, the Activities Director's knowledge of the facility, its programs, and residents was instrumental for the success of groups.

Pre-Group Screening Reflections

One *Older Adults on a Journey* Legacy Group screening session consisted of a Haiku activity that would serve as both an icebreaker and an assessment tool. We were pleasantly surprised to learn that some participants remembered this type of poetry from their high school or college classes. Others remembered teaching it to their own students. The introduction to the Japanese poetry went quickly, and the group was able to complete two or three practice poems easily. Next, we asked the group for a topic and, as if on cue, voices rang out with determination, "cold food." Apparently, the dining room had a reputation for serving their meals cold. We observed *universality* within the group very early as they joked about this shared experience. The resident who served as their representative promised to bring the Haiku to the administration to request change. We were pleased that this introductory session was a success, not only in its own right but also as a catalyst for group *cohesiveness*. These members experienced a sense of belonging and acceptance that would continue to grow and carry them throughout the group experience.

Phase I: Supportive Group Environment and Activity-Based Legacy Exploration (Weeks 1–3)

During the early weeks of the group experience (weeks 1–3), typical legacy activities involve writing from journal prompts; yet many of these older adults required modifications. Using oral storytelling for those who experienced painful arthritic fingers or limited range of motion worked well. Fortunately, we were prepared to adjust so members could participate fully in the group experience.

Another first phase activity that worked well with older adults is a ball activity that offers purpose, guidance, and structure. Light historical prompts are written on the ball: name your first-grade teacher, did you walk to school or get a ride, what was your favorite family vacation as a child, and so on. Group members rolled the ball across the table to another member. The person catching the ball would read the prompt nearest to their right thumb. The stories elicited a variety of emotions and we observed that members listened intently to each shared narrative. Excitement grew when members would reject a prompt and simply select one that they preferred. This behavior resulted in an early group norm, which created a strong foundation for future sharing. Overall, this is an engaging activity that stimulates group members on multiple levels: physical, emotional, and cognitive. As facilitators, we noticed that these group activities offered a window into the familial customs from their past. One Legacy Group comprised seven women and one man, ranging from 55 to 90 years of age. We witnessed generational and gender differences consistent with their generational cohort, and these heterogeneous characteristics served to enrich the group experience.

Attendance to Legacy Group sessions was contingent upon having medical appointments outside the facility, although most managed to preserve group time in their schedule. It was clear that for this cohort, promises made are promises kept, yet another similarity that enhanced the group experience. These older adults were eager to show their independence even though they were living in a residence that provided varying degrees of assistance. Some group members shared that it had been necessary for them to assess their personal belongings and purge varying amounts of furniture, art, books, and memorabilia as they prepared to move into assisted-living quarters. Sadly, some of these older adults moved from large single-family homes where they had raised their family.

The *universality* of their shared experiences was touching and tragic as the painful process of dispersal of their life-long treasures became evident. The *Older Adults on a Journey* Legacy Group experience provided a venue to process these changes. Some members shared a sense of lightness and liberation. Others talked about significant loss. Whichever they claimed, they all had kept something of personal-emotional value (e.g., photographs, letters, coins, jewelry).

Phase II: Personal Legacy Work; Guidance and Support (Weeks 4–10)

Legacy Groups conducted in skilled care facilities with residents who experience short-term memory loss tended to repeatedly tell the same story. We recommend receiving each telling with the same level of anticipation and care while facilitating the group process around legacy exploration and preservation. The repetition may be due to cognitive decline, or it may also be the result of an unconscious life-processing strategy and may offer kindling for a legacy epiphany.

Other group members may tell their story in bits and pieces. One woman, animated and vibrant, thrived on positive energy. Complaints about weather were met with reminders of what they could accomplish indoors. Excuses using physical health were challenged. We were witness to the *installation of hope* in action as she repeatedly encouraged others to look on the brighter side of every day. We would come to learn more about her own story when she shared about her life as a teenage girl conscripted into the Israeli Army. Instead of complaining, finding excuses, or even looking to the good, she opted to keep the story brief, simply sharing that as a citizen of Israel she was required to serve. But as the weeks continued, so too did her story, sharing details about the rigors of training, pride in serving, and descriptions of soldiers who served with her. Whether her memories came to the surface over time or she experienced a sense of safety among her group members is not known. Whichever it was, possibly both, she decided to record those memories for her family by asking her granddaughter to conduct an oral history with her. This *cathartic* retelling served as a *corrective recapitulation of her primary family* as she carefully constructed the way in which she would preserve this long-buried story. We did not hear the finished legacy-taped story, but we never once doubted its completion.

Hands-on activities are as important as writing and oral storytelling or collaging. Selecting appropriate magazines for group members is a key component. For older adults, great choices to foster legacy involve home cooking, classic cars, movies, as well as magazines that depict black and white photos. Members are instructed to select meaningful words and images to create a visual representation of themselves. This is a great activity to build group *cohesion*, especially when facilitators participate. Moving experiences are often shared regarding group members past, their passions, and their hopes and dreams. In one special occasion, a group member residing in a long-term care facility was much younger than the other residents. She needed care due to a stroke that significantly impaired functioning on one side of her body and she required the use of a wheelchair. Her mind, however, was very sharp and she had a quick wit. Initially she wondered about the benefits of joining a Legacy Group (i.e., her physical constraints, difference in age). She did join and was able to use her hands well enough to tear out pictures and words easily. Gluing proved to be more difficult. A woman seated next to her volunteered to assist her. When her collage was completed, she shared her story and her face simply lit up. She was clearly proud of her high-powered career and the energy and passion for her work was conveyed during her storytelling. Group members listened with intensity and interest. They validated her experience and spoke to her with respect and care. Facilitators framed each person's collage and gave them to members to bring back to their rooms so that this legacy project and group experience would be close to them each day.

Phase III: Reflection and Celebration (Weeks 11 and 12)

Reflecting and celebrating are important parts of the termination process. Facilitators offer group members a place and time to reflect, not only their experience as an individual but also as part of a group as well as time to celebrate. At one *Older Adults on a Journey* Legacy Group session, a Wordle was created and given to each group member during the last group session. The Wordle was based on notes kept by the facilitator about each member's legacy: their stories, historical information, and individual characteristics. Individual Wordle's were framed and given to members during the last group session. Members were very touched, felt heard, and seen by the facilitators. One of the oldest males who served as a spokesperson for the group had tears in his eyes as he shared his deep appreciation for this group-ending gift.

As mental health professionals, we are trained to assist group members adapt to life changes. A group member had stopped attending group midway as he had become ill and diagnosed with a terminal illness. On the last day of *Older Adults on a Journey* Legacy Group, the facilitators were able to visit him after the last session of the group experience, as it was conducted in a long-term care facility. He showed us his wall of family photos, many of his memorabilia were in shadow boxes and under the glass top of his coffee table. Apparently, he and his wife had traveled extensively before her death, and he had kept many of the items that they had collected on their travels. We assured him that this is the stuff of legacy. We had a few index cards with us and suggested that he use them to describe each item: when, where, and how you decided to purchase an item and other memories associated with each item. He agreed to *impart information* that would otherwise be lost forever. Certainly, the personal notes describing journeys, cultures, and thoughts could be read and appreciated by his family for generations to come, but we suspected that over the coming days and weeks, he would process his life and legacy.

In their own way, each older adult reflected on their legacy, some with the brevity and speed of a person who wastes no time on emotions, while others more slowly as they revealed memories that their stories evoked. We celebrated each participant's ability to explore and identify their own personal legacy. We believe that each member benefited from the group experience. So too will the generations that enjoy the legacy memories they offered.

References

Cassidy, C. (2017, December 5). *Female veterans feeling underserved by VA*. The National Association of Veteran-Serving Organizations (NAVSO). www.navso.org/news/female-veterans-feeling-underserved-va

Szymendra, S. D. (2016, May 25). *Who is a "Veteran"? Basic eligibility of veterans' benefits*. Congressional Research Service, Analyst in Disability Policy.

8

POTENTIAL AUDIENCES, CHALLENGES, AND SPECIAL CONSIDERATIONS

The Legacy Model was developed to enhance the psychological wellness of veterans and older adults who are interested in exploring and preserving their legacy in a group experience. The development of the Legacy Model was the result of a multiyear community service and research project that offered free wellness groups to interested veterans and older adults. Legacy Groups were conducted and assessed using the Ryff Scale of Psychological Well-Being (Ryff, 2014; Seifert, 2005) to measure the effectiveness of the Legacy Model over a seven-year period. The data were collected exclusively on veterans and older adults aged between 55 and 100+ years. Study results showed the Legacy Group intervention improved psychological well-being for participants, specifically in the areas of Personal Growth and Purpose in Life.

Chapter 8 discusses potential populations that include K–12 settings and college students and staff, persons recovering from loss of a pet, career changes, or friendship seeking, as well as the option for using telehealth delivery of Legacy Groups. Three noteworthy challenges that facilitators may encounter when conducting Legacy Groups, namely, DNA testing results, family secrets, and ethical dilemmas, are discussed. Last, important considerations are highlighted: selection/exclusion criteria and informed consent. Resources are provided to assist facilitators in following the best practices.

Potential Audiences for Legacy Groups

A few years into the project, it became evident that other populations would benefit from a Legacy Group experience. As a result of extensive outreach by the Legacy Team to advertise these groups, other community leaders contacted the Team to inquire about the possibility of adapting the Legacy Model to a

DOI: 10.4324/9781003298168-10

workshop delivery format. This idea was of great interest, that is, the opportunity to explore legacy with other audiences. Given this interest, Legacy Workshops were conducted with college students, food insecure individuals at a community center, and retirees at several Councils on Aging in surrounding communities (Box 8.1). These workshops were delivered in two formats: a onetime two-hour block or a two-meeting format. Legacy topics were selected in collaboration with professional staff who had knowledge and expertise with the population they served. Attendance numbers ranged from as few as five adults in a community center to 40 students at a two-year college. Legacy Workshops received very good reviews from both participants and professional staff.

BOX 8.1   POTENTIAL NEW AUDIENCES

* K–12 settings
* College students
* College/University faculty, staff, administrators
* Recovering from loss of pet, career, friendship

Humes (1994) published an article for school counselors, recommending the use of genealogy as a counseling strategy with students to help foster a sense of identity and enhance self-worth by exploring multiple generations of their ancestors. The author (Humes, 1994) provides various projects for middle and high school students to facilitate this exploration. These projects included conducting oral histories, researching documents online, and visiting public or state libraries and national archives to research records in person. In doing so, students gain research skills, learn about their ancestors' military service, heritage, and the countries their relatives once lived in. Dustin Axe, the Youth Genealogy Curriculum Coordinator at the New England Genealogy Historical Society (New England Genealogy Historical Society, 2021) in Boston, is "creating a national curriculum (grades 4–6) with the goal to make genealogy accessible to all students." This is an exciting project that holds significant psycho-socio-emotional and academic benefits for youths.

Okkiishi (1987) described the value of using career genograms with students as a counseling strategy to explore the careers of their ancestors. The genogram originated with Bowen (1980) and has been used extensively in family therapy over the years. McGoldrick et al. (2008) have published a third edition of *Genograms: Assessment and Intervention*, a comprehensive book for using genograms for understanding family patterns. Reiser (2012) investigated the use of exploring family history to foster college student development. His qualitative study revealed that the participants had increased identity development, enhanced the quality of current relationships, and gave an opportunity to explore spirituality, and learn about shared qualities with their ancestors. The findings from these studies were consistent with the Legacy Team's experience when conducting Legacy Workshops.

Telehealth Legacy Groups

Virtual groups became a necessity during the COVID-19 pandemic as mental health practitioners looked for new ways to connect with students and clients (Pierce et al., 2021). An important distinction to note is that Legacy Groups were designed as a wellness intervention and not a therapy group. As such, these groups lend themselves nicely to an online delivery format. A colleague attended one of our Legacy Group Workshops for mental health professionals at a group conference prior to the COVID-19 pandemic. When the move to online delivery commenced, she decided to teach counseling students in training about the Legacy Model. She reported success mentoring doctoral counseling students while conducting Legacy Groups online with older adults.

Gilbertson (2020) published *Telemental Health: The Essential Guide to Providing Successful Online Therapy*, a comprehensive and helpful resource for practitioners. She offers noteworthy guidance for individuals interested in conducting Legacy Groups using an online delivery format. When conducting online groups with older adults, Gilbertson (2020) recommends using larger visuals to accommodate vision challenges with older adults. Another recommendation when working with older adults with hearing loss online is to recommend headphones designed for hearing impaired individuals. As for cognitive impairment, she recommends limiting the number of steps related to technology to simplify sequences.

Resources continue to grow for practitioners interested in conducting groups online. The Substance Abuse and Mental Health Services Administration (SAMHSA) (2020) created a four-page *Tip Sheet: Group Teletherapy Best Practices, Skills, and Strategies for Providing Virtual Group Psychotherapy* that provides valuable information when conducting online Legacy Groups. Guth et al. (2021) published *Ten Tips for the Facilitation of Virtual Groups* that provides useful tips for all types of group work online: task, psychoeducational, counseling, and therapy groups. Using an online delivery could have the potential to reach out to older adults who have mobility limitations or limited access to transportation.

Potential Challenges

Exploring one's legacy is both exciting and daunting. The journey is likely to involve many ups and downs. Three of the more daunting challenges are noteworthy: DNA testing, family secrets, and ethical dilemmas. DNA testing has exploded in the United States. It is easy, readily available, and inexpensive. Ancestry and 23andMe offer inexpensive testing kits and maintain a registry should you decide to upload your results and view familial DNA matches. As facilitators of Legacy Groups, we have heard our share of DNA test result surprises experienced by group members. Griffeth's memoir, *The Stranger in My Genes* (2016), is a good example about how DNA test results uncovered a family secret that complicated his life. He shares about his interest in genealogy dating back to 2003, and then taking a DNA test in 2012 that rocked his world. Preparing group members for potential surprises helps to reduce the impact associated with such discoveries.

This is a good Segway into the topic of family secrets. Epstein (2019), a marriage and family therapist, identified three types of family secrets that surface for individuals researching family history:

- Individual – a secret held by one person (e.g., a secret affair)
- Internal Family Secrets – a secret at least two persons know (e.g., hiding a date of a marriage)
- Shared Family Secrets – a secret shared only with family members

An important question for facilitators to consider when conducting Legacy Groups is the readiness of members who choose to research their family history. Normalizing about the potential of discovering a family secret often lessens the shock frequently experienced when learning about a secret. In addition, there are many complexities related to sharing family secrets once unearthed. Some of the more common family matters that may emerge along the journey are listed in Box 8.2. It is prudent for group facilitators to acquaint themselves with these topics as they often surface in legacy work.

BOX 8.2 COMMON FAMILY SECRETS THAT MAY BE DISCOVERED

- DNA test results
- Family secrets
- Ethical dilemmas
- Emotional challenges
- Enslaved ancestors
- Adoptions
- Indian war ancestors
- Racial inequities
- Prison records
- Intergenerational oppression or trauma
- Ancestors who were violent or abusive

Walters (2019) published *Ethical Dilemmas in Genealogy*, where she highlights potential ethical dilemmas related to privacy issues, sharing DNA test results, posting data on living persons on the internet or on social media, stealing photos from family trees, and the sharing of family secrets. The International Society of Genetic Genealogy Wiki (2022) has a section devoted to "Ethics, Guidelines and Standards" that is a good resource for Legacy Group facilitators to help navigate ethical dilemmas that may arise during a Legacy Group experience. Moore et al. (2021) wrote a chapter, "Ethical Dilemmas: What Should I do Now?" that provides information and guidance about ethically relevant quandaries and ethical considerations. These are valuable resources to review prior to conducting a Legacy Group.

One of the authors attended the virtual Bowen Center Spring Conference in April of 2021, titled "Unlocking the Mystery of the Family Emotional History." The conference was devoted to ancestral emotional history, healing, and Bowen theory. Workshop presenters offered insights about intergenerational emotional trauma and the family system issues that necessitate therapeutic intervention. As such, screening is an essential step, particularly for potential members of Process-Focused Legacy Groups, as they are designed as wellness groups and not therapy groups aimed to provide individual or family therapy.

Foor (2017), a licensed mental health clinician and spiritual teacher, offers a different perspective for working with ancestor emotional challenges. His book, *Ancestral Medicine*, is devoted to how one can heal intergenerational patterns of pain. Guidance and exercises are provided as well as how to identify and normalize ancestral contact (i.e., synchronicity, dreams). Foor (2017) incorporates both Eastern and Western philosophies when working toward healing dysfunctional family patterns. This book is well suited for those who incorporate the spiritual dimension in their healing journey.

Special Considerations

The development of the Legacy Model was the result of a multiyear community service and research project that offered free wellness groups to interested veterans and older adults. Legacy Groups are wellness groups, not therapy groups. As such, pre-group screening is an essential component to a successful group experience. Both the Process-Focused Legacy Group curriculum and the Activity-Based Legacy Group curriculum were presented in-depth in Part II Legacy Group Curriculum in Action. Pre-group screening with prospective group members was reviewed.

Legacy Group selection criteria are based upon the interest and desire of the potential member to explore their legacy. Yalom and Leszcz contend that exclusion criteria should be based upon the mental health professional's assessment of individuals who are not conducive to group work related to "intellectual, psychological, or interpersonal reasons" (2020, p. 295). Some important considerations for Legacy Group facilitators include prospective group members who have significant brain injury, are actively abusing drugs and/or alcohol, have unresolved trauma, or are unable to embrace diversity: race, religion, gender, ethnicity, or other political views.

Informed consent is an important component when conducting Legacy Groups. There are great resources available to assist practitioners in developing informed consent documents. The ASGW Guiding Principles for Group Work (2021) provides a framework for both assessment practices and for developing informed consent forms that are applicable to the various mental health disciplines. For practitioners interested in conducting online Legacy Groups, Gilbertson (2020) provides Telemental Health Informed Consent samples for assistance in developing your own forms.

As authors, we had the privilege of facilitating Legacy Groups in a variety of settings. Whether group membership consisted of women veterans, community-dwelling older adults, or residents in skilled nursing facilities, each took on an energy and life of its own. We are grateful to have worked with so many lovely people. They taught us to be patience, to embrace life, and seek meaning small and large – mostly about the healing power of legacy.

References

Association for Specialists in Group Work. (2021, May). *ASGW guiding principles for group work*. https://asgw.org/wp-content/uploads/2021/07/ASGW-Guiding-Principles-May-2021.pdf

Bowen, M. (1980). *Key to the genogram*. Georgetown University Hospital.

Epstein, S. (2019). Three types of family secrets and how they drive families apart. *Psychology Today*. www.guides.loc.gov/family-secrets/online-resources

Foor, D. (2017). *Ancestral medicine: Rituals for personal and family healing*. Bear & Company.

Gilbertson, J. (2020). *Telemental health: The essential guide to providing successful online therapy*. PESI Publishing & Media.

Griffeth, B. (2016). *The stranger in my genes*. New England Historic Genealogy Society.

Guth, L. J., Pepper, E. L., Stephens, A. F., Pollard-Kosidowski, B. L., & Garrow, J. (2021). *Ten* tips for the facilitation of virtual groups. *The Journal for Specialists in Group Work*, 46(4), 309–321.

Humes, C. W. (1994). Genealogy: A counseling tool. *The School Counselor*, 41(4).

The International Society of Genetic Genealogy Wiki. (2022). *Ethics, guidelines and standards*. https://isogg.org/wiki/Ethics,_guidelines_and_standards

McGoldrick, M., Gerson, R., & Shellenberger, S. (2008). *Genograms: Assessment and intervention*. W.W. Norton & Company.

Moore, S., Rosenthal, D., & Robinson, R. (2021). *Ethical dilemmas: What should I do now?* Routledge, Taylor and Francis Group.

New England Genealogy Historical Society. (2021). *Curriculum pilot program*. https://american ancestors.org/curriculum-pilot-program

Okkiishi, R. W. (1987). The genogram as a tool in career counseling. *Journal of Counseling & Development*, 66, 139–143.

Pierce, B. S., Perrin, B. P., Tyler, C. M., McKee, G. B., & Watson, J. D. (2021). The COVID-19 telepsychology revolution: A national study of pandemic-based changes in U.S. mental health care delivery. *American Psychologist, 76*(1), 14–25. https://doi.org/10.1037/amp0000722

Reiser, M. L. (2012). *Exploring genealogical roots and family history and their influence on college student development: A qualitative study* [Dissertation, Brigham Young University, Pro-Quest Dissertation Publications].

Ryff, C. D. (2014). Psychological well-being revisited: Advances in the science and practice of eudaimonia. *Psychotherapy and Psychosomatics, 83*, 10–28. www.jstor.org/stable/48516513

Seifert, T. (2005). *The Ryff scales of psychological well-being.* Center of Inquiry at Wabash College. https://centerofinquiry.org/uncategorized/ryff-scales-of-psychological-well-being/

Substance Abuse and Mental Health Services Administration (SAMHSA). (2020). *Tip sheet: Group teletherapy best practices, skills, and strategies for providing virtual group psychotherapy.* https://mhttcnetwork.org/sites/default/files/2020-08/MHTTC_TelehealthInfo Sheet2_GroupTelehealth_FINAL.pdf

Walters, P. (2019). *Ethical dilemmas in genealogy.* www.amazon.com/Ethical-Dilemmas-Genealogy-Penny_Walters-ebook/dp/B07Ry25KJX

Yalom, I. D. & Leszcz, M. (2020). *The theory and practice of group psychotherapy* (6th ed.). Basic Books.

APPENDIX I

Legacy Project Ideas

A list of projects Legacy Group members have used to explore and/or preserve their legacy is provided next. They are listed alphabetically and include a brief description.

Collaging

Webster's *New World Dictionary* defines a collage as "an art form in which bits of objects, as newspaper, cloth, pressured flowers, etc. are pasted together on a surface in incongruous relationship for their symbolic or suggestive effect" (p. 273). Legacy projects often incorporate historical memorabilia (e.g., photographs, news clippings, popular culture items, receipts, personal artifacts).

Family Cookbook

Sharing and preserving recipes can serve to connect family members while living, as well as to their ancestors. Sharing food together is a great way to enhance relationships. Creating a family cookbook bonds people around culture, important holidays, or celebrations, and connects family members across generations. It is easily collected, preserved, and shared.

Family History Crafts

There are endless craft ideas available either to create a craft yourself or have it made by a company specializing in the type of craft desired. Some of the more popular crafts include having photos placed on clothing or a mug, coasters, ornaments, pillows, or framing a thumbprint, fingerprint, or handprints of family members. Visiting a craft store or searching online oftentimes sparks creative ideas.

Genealogy Research

Francois Weil (2013) wrote *Family Trees: A History of Genealogy in America*. He offers a broad definition of genealogy: "[T]he science of family relationships and lineages or more broadly as a personal interest in one's forebears" (p. 2). For some, their interest lies in researching their family tree. Others want to learn about the lives of their ancestors (e.g., stories, challenges, acquire photographs, connect with living relatives). With the advent of technology, individuals can conduct research from the comfort of their home using Family Search, American Ancestry, or Ancestry. As not all family information is available online, more traditional research methods continue to unveil a wealth of information. Visiting cemeteries, National Archives, local city/town halls to view vital records, and organizations that have research facilities like the New England Historic Genealogy Society continue to be invaluable sources of ancestral and historical material.

Journaling

The Webster's *New World Dictionary* defines a journal as "a daily record of happenings, a diary." When conducting an internet search, various websites state evidence that journaling began around 167 BC. There are numerous reasons people journal: to record thoughts and feelings each day, to deepen one's sense of self and values, to sort through problems, or to leave a written legacy. Ira Progoff wrote *At a Journal Workshop*, which is about intensive journaling that is used to tap into one's inner wisdom and for personal renewal. Journaling may be kept confidential or written for others to view.

Lineage-Based Service Membership

Lineage-based organizations and societies offer membership to individuals who can prove that they are a direct descendant. This is a way to honor your heritage and ancestors. Some examples are DAR, The Huguenot Society of America, The Mayflower Society, and the Sons of the American Revolution. Wikipedia provides an extensive list member-based societies at https://en.wikipedia.org/wiki/List_of_hereditary_and_lineage_organizations.

Memoir Writing

Natalie Goldberg (2007) developed *Old Friend from Far Away: The Practice of Writing Memoir* as a guide for working on a memoir. She provides reflective exercises to assist the individuals in exploring memories and developing the narrative. There are numerous such guides for novices and experienced writers. Memoirs can be written as a journey and be kept personal, shared with family, or published for a wider audience.

Memory Blanket

Making quilts has been traced back to medieval time. They are often made of scraps of material oftentimes from pieces of worn clothing. A memory blanket is theme-based. Some individuals have used a quilt service to place images of grand-children on the blanket and given to grandparents as a gift. There are endless themes used for creating memory blankets: family photos, favorite vacation, and honoring military service are but a few. The blanket can be handcrafted, created by a professional quilter, or constructed from an online service.

Memory Decoupage Box

Creating a keepsake to store letters, pictures, and objects that are mementos from family members and significant relationships is an easy project. The decoupage box is often the size of a shoe box and is decorated with newsprint, photos, or anything personally symbolic. Oftentimes it is created with the intent of giving it as a gift to a special person. Sometimes it is given after completion of a significant accomplishment (i.e., graduation, military boot camp).

Oral History

Flekke (2011) published *Telling Our Stories, Oral and Family History*. The author states that oral history began as oral tradition, the passing down of informa-tion from generation to generation (Flekke, 2011). There are a number of organizations that conduct and collect oral histories. Two examples are the Worcester Women's *Oral History Project* that records and shares the personal histories of women from the Worcester, Massachusetts, or the Veterans History Project where the US government collects and preserves written, audio, and/ or video recordings. A popular method is more informal where an individual can record information or stories about their legacy. One way to conduct an oral history is to create a series of questions that are asked with relatives; as such, multiple persons responding to similar questions are interviewed and preserved.

Photograph Albums, Books, or Displays

Photographs help preserve people, places, and memories in time. Creating digital albums; photo memoir books; and theme pieces for family members, friends, and other loved ones leaves a lasting memory. There are various ways to display photos: a display wall in your home, using precut picture frames, or creating decorative artifacts to hold a special photograph.

Poetry

"Poetry is the spontaneous overflow of powerful feelings; it takes its origin from emotion recollected in tranquility" (Wadsworth Foundation). Writing poetry can serve to convey meaning and deep emotions as well as can be passed down through generations. A type of poem often used during the group experience is Haiku. The ancient Japanese word for poem is *renga*, which is beautifully translated into "lined songs," is the origin of Haiku. A *renga* has a root of 17 syllables that is presented in three lines. Similar to a chain with interlocking links, the first line has five syllables, the second line has seven syllables, and the third line has five syllables. The *renga* is preceded or followed by 14 syllables, two lines of seven syllables each. The *tanka* (lines containing 5–7–5–7–7 syllables) was a ninth- to twelfth-century poem in which one person wrote the first three lines (5–7–5) and then another person completed the last two lines (7–7). Each couplet or tercet produces a poem itself. An example of a Haiku:

> *Embrace legacy*
> *Sweet memories and stories*
> *Personal meaning*
>   – Victoria L. Bacon

Scrapbooking

A scrapbook can be created for endless reasons: to preserve photos, recipes, newspaper articles, awards, tickets, and so on. Some scrapbooks are designed to tell a story or created to document a time in history using various pieces of memorabilia. A scrapbook is easy to make and the books are often inexpensive, and sold at a number of local stores or online with the option to design your own cover.

Shadow Box

A shadow box is a glassed front case that is used to protect, preserve, and display items. The shadow box displays personal artifacts in a three-dimensional collage manner that creates a visual representation of something memorable about an individual. It can also be used to make large collections smaller, saving only the favorite pieces (e.g., jewelry, handkerchiefs, coins, medals, baseball cards).

Writing a Family History

A popular exploration and preservation method is writing a family history. There are numerous published guidebooks available that provide step-by-step instructions and provide guidance on the process of writing your family history. Sharon DeBartolo published *You Can Write Your Family History*, which provides readers with seven potential genres for family history writing: (1) reference genealogy, (2) genealogical narratives, (3) life story writing, (4) family history narratives, (5) family history memoir, (6) edited letters and diaries, and (7) fictional family sagas based on truth. Family histories can be self-published or copied and distributed to family members.

APPENDIX II
Legacy Group Resources

Akeret, R. U., & Klein, D. M. (1991). *Family tales, family wisdom: How to gather the stories of a lifetime and share them with your family*. Morrow.

Anthony, M. (2009). *Mass casualties: A young medic's true story of death, deception, and dishonor in Iraq*. Adams Media.

Berkeley, E. P. (2000). *At grandmother's table: Women write about food, life, and the enduring bond between grandmothers and granddaughters*. Fairview Press.

Browder, L., & Pflaeging, S. (2010). *When Janey comes marching home: Portraits of women combat veterans*. University of North Carolina Press.

Carmack, S. D. (2003). *You can write your family history*. Betterway Books.

Colletta, J. P. (2000). *Only a few bones: A true account of Rolling Fork tragedy and its aftermath*. Direct Descent.

Craig, H. T. (1991). *A priceless legacy: An album of memories for future generations*. Banyan Tree Press.

Croom, E. A. (1995). *Unpuzzling your past: A basic guide to genealogy* (3rd ed.). Betterway Books.

Elgin, D., & LeDrew, C. (2001). *Living legacies: How to write, illustrate, and share your life stories*. Conari Press.

Field, V., Thompson, K., & Bolton, G. (2011). *Writing routes: A resource handbook of therapeutic writing*. Jessica Kingsley.

Flekke, M. M. (2011). *Telling our stories: Oral and family history: A bibliography* (5th ed.). Heritage Books.

Foor, D. (2017). *Ancestral medicine: Rituals for personal and family healing*. Bear & Company.

Freed, R. (2012). *The legacy workbook for the busy woman* (2nd ed.). Minerva Press.

Fulford, D. G. (2000). *One memory at a time: Inspiration and advice for writing your family story*. Doubleday.

Goldberg, N. (2007). *Old friend from far away: The practice of writing memoir*. Atria Books.

Greene, B., & Fulford, D. G. (1993). *To our children's children: Preserving family histories for generations to come*. Doubleday.

Hoff, H. B. (2002). *Genealogical writing in the 21st century: A guide to register style and more.* New England Historic Genealogical Society.

Knox, J., & Knox, T. (2005). *Letters from 'Nam: A family memoir.* Author House.

Laumann, S., & Fraser, S. (2014). *Unsinkable: My untold story.* HarperCollins Canada.

Leibovitz, M., & Solomon, L. (1993). *Legacies.* HarperCollins.

Luttrell, M., & Robinson, P. (2007). *Lone survivor: The eyewitness account of operation redwing and the lost heroes of SEAL team 10.* Little, Brown and Company.

Merriam-Webster. (2003). Litmus test. In *Merriam-Webster's collegiate dictionary* (11th ed., p. 727).

Matos, G. (2011). *Shattered glass: The story of a marine embassy guard.* Two Harbors Press.

McClure, R. R. (2004). *Digitizing your family history: Easy methods for preserving your heirloom documents, photos, home movies and more in a digital format.* Family Tree Books.

McCord, K. (2012). *My CIA: A memoir.* Telling Our Stories Press.

Norman, E. M. (1999). *We band of angels: The untold story of American nurses trapped on Bataan by the Japanese.* Random House.

Progoff, I. (1975). *At a journal workshop: The basic text and guide for using the intensive journal.* Dialogue House Library.

Putney, W. W. (2001). *Always faithful: A memoir of the Marine dogs of WWII.* Free Press.

Roberts, L., Buchanan, M., & Roberts, R. (2012). *My story, my song: Mother-daughter reflections on life and faith.* Upper Room Books.

Rose, C. (2004). *Courthouse research for family historians: Your guide to genealogical treasures.* CR Publications.

Rosenbluth, V. (1990). *Keeping family stories alive: A creative guide to taping your family life & lore.* Hartley & Marks.

Slan, J. C. (1999). *Scrapbook storytelling: Save family stories and memories with photos, journaling and your own creativity.* E. F. G. Publishers.

Taylor, D. (2005). *Letters to my children: A father passes on his values.* Bog Walk Press.

Taylor, D. (2011). *Creating a spiritual legacy: How to share your stories, values, and wisdom.* Brazos Press.

Taylor, M. A. (1999). *Through the eyes of your ancestors.* Houghton Mifflin.

Taylor, M. A. (2013). *Family photo detective: Learn how to find genealogy clues in old photos and solve family photo mysteries.* Family Tree Books.

Thorpe, H. (2014). *Soldier girls: The battles of three women at home and at war.* Scribner.

Wakefield, R. (1989). *What did you do in the war, grandma? An oral history of Rhode Island women during World War II.* Linda P. Wood and Judi Scott.

Weil, F. (2013). *Family trees: A history of genealogy in America.* Harvard University Press.

INDEX

Note: Page numbers in *italics* indicate a figure and page numbers in **bold** indicate a table on the corresponding page.

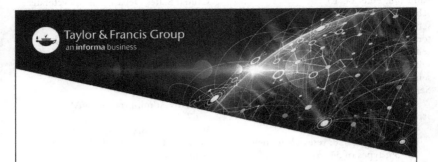

Taylor & Francis Group
an **informa** business

Taylor & Francis eBooks

www.taylorfrancis.com

A single destination for eBooks from Taylor & Francis
with increased functionality and an improved user
experience to meet the needs of our customers.

90,000+ eBooks of award-winning academic content in
Humanities, Social Science, Science, Technology, Engineering,
and Medical written by a global network of editors and authors.

TAYLOR & FRANCIS EBOOKS OFFERS:

A streamlined
experience for
our library
customers

A single point
of discovery
for all of our
eBook content

Improved
search and
discovery of
content at both
book and
chapter level

REQUEST A FREE TRIAL
support@taylorfrancis.com

 Routledge
Taylor & Francis Group

 CRC Press
Taylor & Francis Group